HERBAL BIOHACKING FOR WOMEN

NATURAL & ANCIENT PLANT REMEDIES FOR
HORMONE BALANCE, MENTAL CLARITY, STRESS
REDUCTION, IMMUNE SUPPORT AND GRACEFUL
AGING

SAGE O'REILLY

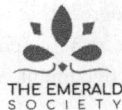

THE EMERALD
SOCIETY

LEAVE A REVIEW

Don't forget to share the love and **leave your
<u>Amazon review</u>** for:

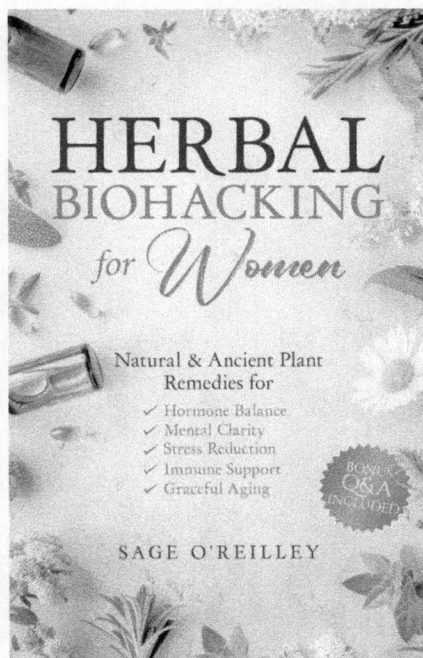

HERBAL
BIOHACKING
for Women

Natural & Ancient Plant
Remedies for

✓ Hormone Balance
✓ Mental Clarity
✓ Stress Reduction
✓ Immune Support
✓ Graceful Aging

BONUS
Q&A
INCLUDED

SAGE O'REILLEY

THE COMPLETE
CORTISOL
DETOX
HANDBOOK

3
BOOKS
IN 1

A Practical Guide &
Workbook for Balancing
Hormones, Regulating
Emotions, Healing Your Gut,
Reducing Inflammation and
Managing stress

30+
RECIPES
INCLUDED

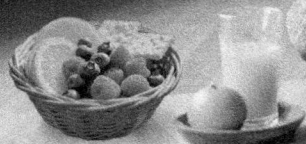

SAGE O'REILLEY

CONTENTS

PREFACE

Dearest reader,

Here's the truth.

I didn't set out to write a book that would flirt shamelessly with the boundaries of biohacking, herbalism, and hormonal rebellion. As a holistic health specialist, I was simply doing what I'd always done: working with women, listening deeply, and offering support founded in science and nature.

But then something shifted. More and more women—smart, accomplished, exhausted—were sitting across from me asking the same questions in slightly different voices: *Why am I doing everything "right" and still feeling off? Why is my energy tanking, my mood swinging, and my sleep acting like an unreliable ex?* The answers weren't in a prescription pad or a 10-minute consultation. They were deeper, messier, more beautifully complex, and they were begging for a new kind of conversation.

Initially, this book was going to be a sweet, grounded guide to natural herbs and homemade remedies. Think Pinterest boards, mason jars, and elderberry syrup made with love. But somewhere between infusions and elixirs, a louder, sassier voice emerged, one that wasn't here for the soft-glow lifestyle fluff. This voice wanted results. It wanted to sleep through the night, wake up with energy that didn't come in a mug, and feel alive and thriving in a body that was no longer twenty (and didn't want to be, thank you very much).

That voice? She wrote this book.

So yes, we'll still be playing with plants. But this time, we're doing it with strategy. While parts of this book *do* cover the basics—because, truthfully, most of the women I work with haven't yet had the pleasure of stepping into the world of herbal medicine—there's a deeper layer here, and that's where the real magic happens. This isn't just an herbal handbook; it's a guided entry into the world of herbal biohacking. It's for women, potentially life yourself, who've lived long enough to know that the status quo doesn't cut it. It's for women who are done being told to "just relax" while their hormones throw impromptu dance parties at 3 AM. It's for the ones who know that true health isn't about simply getting by. It's about reclaiming your fire, your focus, and your fierce with a little attitude and a whole lot of intention.

If you've read *The Complete Cortisol Detox Handbook*, then you already know I don't believe in quick fixes or cookie-cutter advice. What I do believe in is the beautiful complexity of women's bodies, the underestimated power of plants, and the magic that happens when we put the two together with purpose. This book is a natural extension of that detox journey, expanding the conversation into a fuller, richer, dare-I-say sexier territory of vitality, hormone harmony, and whole-body wellness.

So, here's what you can expect: a little science, a little sass, and a whole lot of practical magic. We'll explore adaptogens that help your body chill out without checking out, and we'll meet botanical allies that know how to coax your inner fire back to life, without burning you out in the process. Along the way, you'll discover powerful, plant-based ways to hack your hormones—not just for physical balance, but for mental clarity, sharper focus, and emotional equilibrium.

This book is for the wild-hearted, wise women who know that aging is not a decline, but an evolution and a privilege. And herbs? They're not just weeds or window dressings. They're our allies. They've been waiting—quietly, patiently—for us to remember their power.

Let's get into it. Your next chapter starts now, and it smells faintly of lavender and rebellion.

— *Sage*

HERBAL HEALING

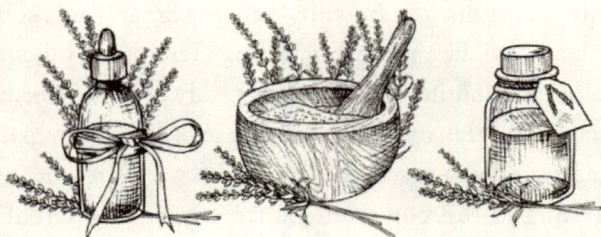

" Nature provides us with everything we need to restore
balance and harmony within ourselves.

- ALCHEMY OF HERBS

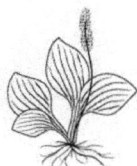

INTRODUCTION

I n the quiet corners of a bustling city, a woman finds solace in the gentle leaves of her rooftop garden. Her journey began with a simple cup of chamomile tea, which not only soothed her nerves but sparked a curiosity that transformed her life. Her story isn't uncommon; in fact, it reflects a growing trend where more and more of us are reawakening to the power of nature, turning to herbal remedies not just as a supplementary choice, but as a primary avenue to enhance well-being.

In recent years, a significant shift has been observed, with 38% of adults in the U.S. now incorporating some form of herbal medicine into their health care regimen. Meanwhile, my own path into the world of herbal healing began over a decade ago, during a particularly stressful time in my life when conventional medicine seemed more about managing symptoms than fostering healing. A serendipitous encounter with a naturopath opened my eyes to the potency of plants. Propelled by this revelation, I pursued a deeper understanding, eventually diverging my career and life path towards mastering naturopathy. My commitment has grown from personal use to sharing what I've learned with others, driven by the conviction that nature offers some of the most reliable tools for health and wellness.

This unique handbook was crafted to demystify the process of using herbs to maintain and enhance health. It is designed to be a clear, practical tool that spans the spectrum from introducing beginners to the fundamentals of herbal medicine, to enriching the repertoire of those of us with more in-depth knowledge. It bridges age-old herbal traditions and modern scientific findings, offering a balanced perspective that respects and utilizes both.

Therefore, this book is for those who seek not only to understand but to apply the principles of herbal healing in everyday life. Whether you are just starting out or looking to deepen your existing practice, here you will find information that is both accessible and actionable.

Structured to facilitate ease of understanding, these pages include simple recipes, insightful anecdotes, and the latest research, ensuring that you have a well-rounded grasp of each topic discussed.

So, as you prepare to transform your approach to well-being, let this be your call to action to embrace natural health by integrating herbal remedies into your life. I encourage you to engage with each recipe and tip, and to embrace a more holistically-informed path to health. I also recommend keeping a journal of your experiences. This return to nature - to yourself - is a beautiful path of learning and self-discovery.

Welcome to your journey back to the roots, where healing, growth, and holistic wellness await.

ONE

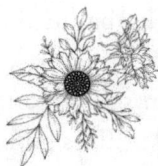

BIOHACKING BASICS FOR WOMEN

What is Herbal Biohacking?

L et's clear something up right out of the gate: biohacking doesn't mean turning your kitchen into a chemistry lab or swapping your soul for a Fitbit. It means getting curious—and strategic—about how your body works and how to support it naturally so it works *better*. When we add herbs into the mix, we're not just hacking—we're healing with intention.

Herbal biohacking consists of using plant-based tools such as adaptogens, nervines, hormone-balancing herbs, nootropics, and more to gently fine-tune our internal systems. We're not here to override the body's wisdom. We're here to partner with it. Think of it as giving your hormones a spa day, your nervous system a warm hug, and your brain a double espresso made of ginkgo and lion's mane.

But here's the twist: women's bodies aren't just smaller versions of men's (*obviously*). We're rhythmic, cyclical, and highly responsive to subtle changes. Which means that *our* biohacking processes looks different, especially after 40, when the rules start to shift in ways no one warned us about in health class.

Why Biohacking After 40 Is Different

Here's the truth: if you've crossed the fabulous 4-0 threshold, your body is writing a new manual (and you probably didn't get a copy).

What used to work—cutting carbs, going hard at spin class, staying up past 11 without consequences—suddenly... doesn't. That's not you failing. That's biology evolving.

Around this age, your estrogen and progesterone begin their peri-menopausal rollercoaster ride. (Please keep arms and legs inside the vehicle at all times.) Meanwhile, cortisol, your primary stress hormone, is like, "Hey, let's make this interesting!" and starts overreacting to, well, everything. Add to that a metabolism that's taking more naps than it used to, and a brain occasionally wrapped in brain fog, and it's no wonder you feel off.

Biohacking in this chapter of life is about supporting *adaptation*. Your body isn't breaking, it's transitioning. And herbs, when used wisely, can help guide you through it with more clarity, more calm, and fewer nights staring at the ceiling at 3 AM wondering if you left the oven on in 1998.

This is the moment to stop trying to "bounce back" and start tuning in. To embrace herbal biohacking not as a rescue mission, but as a reclamation.

Hormones 101: Your Body's Key Players

Let's have a quick look at the main hormones that regulate your body.

ESTROGEN: The star of the show. Keeps your skin supple, bones strong, brain sharp, and mood relatively sane. During perimenopause, it fluctuates wildly, sometimes high, sometimes ghosting you like a bad date.

. . .

PROGESTERONE: The calming, grounding presence. It helps you sleep, keeps anxiety in check, and balances estrogen's diva energy. It's usually the first to exit the stage in your 40s, which is why insomnia and irritability often show up before a single hot flash.

CORTISOL: Your stress responder. When balanced, it helps you wake up energized and handle life's chaos. When imbalanced, it's behind the belly fat, brain fog, sugar cravings, and "Why did I just cry over a yogurt commercial?" moments.

INSULIN: The sugar whisperer. It manages your blood sugar levels and energy. As estrogen drops, insulin resistance can creep in, meaning your body stores fat more easily, especially around the midsection.

THYROID HORMONES: The tempo-keepers of metabolism. They regulate how fast or slow your body ticks. And they're sensitive little things, often impacted by stress, sleep, toxins, and inflammation. Thyroid sluggishness is common in midlife, often mistaken for "just getting older."

WHEN THESE HORMONES are working together, it leads to a peaceful, energy-rich life. Herbal biohacking is your toolkit for tuning these back to harmony—naturally, gently, and without giving up wine or joy (unless you want to).

What Happens in Midlife (and Why It Feels Like a Plot Twist)

By the time you reach your 40s and beyond, your body starts shifting in noticeable ways. You may feel tired more often, gain weight even without changing your habits, experience mood swings, or find it harder to concentrate. This isn't just "aging." These are often signs of hormonal shifts, inflammation, and changes in how your body processes stress, food, and sleep.

Let's break it down.

1. Fluctuating Hormones

ESTROGEN, progesterone, and other key hormones don't decline steadily. They fluctuate—up one day, down the next—which creates physical and emotional instability. One week, you might feel sharp and energetic. The next, you're exhausted and irritable for no clear reason. These ups and downs are common during perimenopause and can continue into menopause if not supported.

2. Increased Stress Response

YOUR BODY BECOMES MORE reactive to stress. Cortisol, your main stress hormone, may stay elevated longer than it used to. Chronic stress keeps your nervous system in a constant state of alert, which can lead to poor sleep, increased belly fat, food cravings, and even memory issues.

3. Metabolic Changes

YOUR METABOLISM SLOWS DOWN. Muscle mass gradually declines, and your body may become less efficient at burning calories. This is partly due to declining estrogen and thyroid activity, and partly due to reduced physical activity or nutrient absorption.

4. Blood Sugar Sensitivity

As ESTROGEN DROPS, your body becomes more sensitive to carbohydrates. Foods you once handled easily may now cause blood sugar spikes, followed by crashes, leaving you tired, moody, or craving sugar soon after eating.

5. Digestive and Gut Health Shifts

YOUR DIGESTION MAY ALSO CHANGE. You might notice more bloating, gas, or irregularity. Hormones influence gut motility and enzyme production, and stress can interfere with how well you digest and absorb nutrients.

6. Sleep Disruptions

FALLING asleep or staying asleep can become more difficult. Lower progesterone affects relaxation and melatonin production, while high cortisol keeps you awake. The result is lighter, more fragmented sleep, and a harder time recovering from daily stress.

7. Mood and Mental Clarity

FLUCTUATIONS IN ESTROGEN and progesterone affect neurotransmitters like serotonin and dopamine, which influence mood and mental focus. You may feel more anxious, depressed, forgetful, or easily overwhelmed, not because you're "losing it," but because your brain chemistry is in flux.

. . .

THESE SHIFTS ARE REAL, not imagined. They're also not signs of weakness or failure. They're your body's way of signaling that it needs a new kind of support. What worked in your 20s and 30s won't necessarily work now—and that's not a bad thing. It's just a different stage with different needs.

Rebalancing Naturally: Basic Hacks

Before we fully immerse ourselves into the world of herbal health, let's take a look at a few important considerations when it comes to biohacking an aging body.

You don't need to overhaul your entire life to feel better. But you *do* need to give your body what it's asking for now. That means tuning into your hormones, metabolism, and nervous system, and supporting them with consistent, foundational strategies. Nothing extreme. Nothing punishing. Just smart, effective changes that work with your biology.

1. Nourish First, Don't Restrict

Forget cutting everything out. Start by adding in what your body needs most right now:

- **Protein:** Aim for 20–30 grams per meal. Protein helps balance blood sugar, supports lean muscle, and improves hormone metabolism.
- **Healthy fats:** Avocados, nuts, seeds, olive oil, fatty fish. These support hormone production and reduce inflammation.
- **Fiber:** Crucial for gut health, blood sugar control, and estrogen detoxification. Think vegetables, legumes, and flaxseed.

- **Complex carbs:** Don't fear carbs—fear *unbalanced* carbs. Prioritize whole grains, root veggies, and legumes paired with protein or fat to avoid sugar crashes.

Food is not just fuel, it's information. What you eat tells your body how to function.

2. Balance Blood Sugar—Non-Negotiable

This is one of the fastest ways to feel more stable—physically and mentally. Blood sugar highs and lows can mimic anxiety, fatigue, and irritability.

Start here:

- Don't skip meals.
- Include protein and fat at every meal.
- Avoid naked carbs (like plain toast or fruit without a protein/fat).
- Walk after meals to improve glucose control.
- Even minor tweaks can make a big difference within days.

3. Support Your Stress Response

Your nervous system is not meant to be "on" all the time. If cortisol stays elevated, it disrupts sleep, digestion, hormones, and fat storage.

Build daily calm, not just weekend escapes:

- Breathe: Deep belly breathing for 3–5 minutes lowers cortisol fast.
- Adaptogens: Herbs like ashwagandha, rhodiola, and holy basil help your body adapt to stress.
- Boundaries: Learn to say "no" without guilt. Energy conservation is hormonal therapy.

4. Prioritize Sleep Like It's Medicine

Because it is. Hormone repair, fat metabolism, memory, and mood are all linked to your sleep quality.

Sleep basics that matter:

- Consistent bedtime and wake time.
- Cool, dark room.
- No screens 60 minutes before bed (or at least use blue-light blockers).
- Magnesium glycinate or a calming herbal tea (like chamomile or lemon balm) to unwind.

If sleep is off, everything else becomes harder to fix.

5. Exercise Isn't Optional

IF THERE's one lifestyle shift that can impact *every* system in your body, it's movement. As estrogen declines, staying active becomes even more critical for hormone balance, metabolism, mental clarity, and emotional health. Midlife is when many women begin to lose muscle, slow their metabolism, and feel more fatigued. Regular movement helps reverse all of that.

Why it matters now more than ever:

- **Strength training (2–4x/week):** Prevents muscle loss, supports metabolism, improves insulin sensitivity, and protects your bones (estrogen loss increases fracture risk).
- **Cardiovascular exercise:** Supports heart health, brain function, mood, and fat metabolism. Walking, cycling, swimming, dancing—it all counts.
- **Mobility and flexibility work:** Yoga, Pilates, and dynamic stretching reduce injury risk, ease joint stiffness, and support nervous system regulation.
- **Short movement bursts:** Even 10–15 minutes can improve blood sugar, lower cortisol, and shift your mood.

Consistency is the secret weapon—not perfection. The more you move, the better your body processes hormones, burns fat, digests food, and recovers from stress.

It's one of the most powerful tools you have to biohack aging, naturally and effectively.

6. Ditch the "Just Deal With It" Mentality

Symptoms are messages, not life sentences. You're not meant to feel tired, foggy, bloated, or anxious every day. Midlife is not a slow decline—it's a recalibration. When you give your body the right tools, it adapts. You just need to stop fighting it, and start listening.

TWO

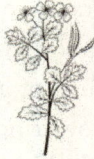

FUNDAMENTALS OF HERBAL
MEDICINE

Have you ever wondered how a simple plant can change the way your body works or heals? This chapter is where we unfold the magic and science of herbal medicine, a practice as ancient as humanity itself but as relevant as any modern medical discovery. Here, you will begin to see herbs not just as plants or ingredients in your kitchen but as powerful tools for healing and well-being. We will explore the roots of herbal medicine, understand the science behind it, and appreciate its role in different cultures and modern healthcare. This knowledge isn't just academic; it's a way to empower you to make informed decisions about your health and integrate age-old wisdom into your everyday life.

The Roots of Herbal Medicine: A Journey from Past to Present

The story of herbal medicine is as old as civilization itself. Ancient texts from Egypt, China, and India describe medicinal uses of plants that are still used today. For instance, the Ebers Papyrus from Egypt, dating back to 1550 BCE, lists over 850 plant medicines, including garlic for heart conditions and aloe vera for skin health. Similarly,

Ayurveda from India and Traditional Chinese Medicine have rich traditions of using herbs to balance the body's energies and promote health. These practices were not just medical treatments but a way of life, integrating spiritual, physical, and mental health.

The evolution of herbal medicine through the centuries demonstrates its efficacy and resilience. In medieval Europe, monks in monasteries kept elaborate herb gardens and translated Arabic medical texts that preserved much of ancient herbal knowledge. The Renaissance period saw the flowering of herbalism anew with the publication of herbals that made knowledge about medicinal plants more accessible. Despite the rise of synthetic drugs in the 20th century, herbal medicine has experienced a resurgence as people seek safe, natural, and holistic approaches to health care.

Scientific Foundation

UNDERSTANDING how herbs work in the body involves a bit of science. Phytochemistry, the study of chemicals found in plants, explains how plants produce these compounds to protect themselves from pests, disease, and environmental stresses. These same plant chemicals, including alkaloids, flavonoids, and essential oils, can benefit human health. For example, the salicin in willow bark is a precursor to aspirin's active ingredient, acetylsalicylic acid, which is widely used for pain relief.

Pharmacognosy, another key scientific field, involves the study of medicinal drugs derived from plants and other natural sources. This discipline has allowed scientists to understand how plant compounds interact with human biology, leading to the development of numerous medications. However, unlike synthetic drugs, herbal remedies offer a complex mixture of ingredients that work together synergistically, often producing fewer side effects and promoting balance within the body.

Modern Integration

TODAY, herbal medicine is gaining ground within the scientific community and public health spheres, evidenced by increasing clinical trials and the integration of herbal protocols in holistic medical practices. Hospitals and medical schools are beginning to embrace these ancient practices, with courses in herbal medicine offered alongside conventional curricula. This integration is supported by a growing body of research that validates the efficacy of herbal treatments in a variety of conditions, from chronic illnesses like arthritis to mental health issues such as depression and anxiety.

The World Health Organization (WHO) estimates that 80% of the world's population uses herbal medicine for some aspect of primary health care. This statistic reflects the global reach of herbal medicine, as well as its potential to complement conventional medical treatments, leading to more comprehensive, accessible, and personalized care.

Cultural Appreciation

HERBAL MEDICINE IS NOT JUST about the herbs themselves but the wisdom of the cultures that have used them for centuries. Each culture brings a unique perspective on how to use plants for healing. For example, Native American healing practices, Ayurveda, and Traditional Chinese Medicine each have distinct methods and philosophies but share a common respect for nature's healing powers.

Recognizing and respecting these diverse traditions is crucial for a truly holistic approach to health. It involves understanding the cultural significance of certain plants and healing practices, which can deepen one's appreciation and effectiveness of herbal treatments. In today's global village, integrating these diverse practices with sensitivity and respect can lead to more effective and meaningful health outcomes for everyone involved.

As we explore these foundations, we can aim to remember that this knowledge is not just historical or theoretical. It's a living, breathing part of everyday wellness that you can tap into to enhance your own health and that of your family.

Deciphering the Language of Plants: A Glossary for Beginners

Navigating the world of herbal medicine can sometimes feel like learning a new language. From tinctures to decoctions, each term carries a depth of tradition and scientific backing that can transform your understanding and practice of herbal remedies. Let's begin by demystifying some of these essential terms, making them accessible and useful for your everyday life. Understanding these will enhance your knowledge, as well as empower you to apply this ancient natural wisdom effectively in caring for yourself and your loved ones.

A tincture is perhaps one of the most common herbal preparations you might come across. It involves extracting the medicinal properties of a plant using alcohol or vinegar. The process results in a concentrated liquid that delivers the benefits of the herb efficiently into the body. For instance, a few drops of a lavender tincture might be just what you need to ease anxiety or help you drift off to sleep. Decoctions, on the other hand, involve simmering tougher plant materials like roots or bark in water to extract their vital compounds. This method is ideal for creating potent remedies from hardy materials that need more coaxing to release their beneficial properties, much like making a robust stock in your kitchen.

Infusions are another cornerstone of herbal medicine, similar to brewing a cup of tea but often with a therapeutic intent. By steeping leaves or flowers in hot water, their medicinal qualities are imparted into the water, creating a gentle yet effective remedy for various ailments. For example, an infusion of chamomile flowers can be a soothing treatment for an upset stomach or a stressful day.

Then there are salves, which are thick, ointment-like preparations made by infusing herbs into oils and then thickening them with beeswax. They are applied externally to heal skin issues, wounds, or inflammations. Think of a salve as a protective barrier that carries healing right to where it's needed, soothing a burn or an irritating rash with nature's touch.

The importance of botanical nomenclature - the use of scientific names for herbs - is an important practice in the world of natural remedies. Although at times it may seem like academic pedantry, it is important to understand that using exact terms is vital to ensure clarity and safety in herbalism. Common names can be misleading or duplicated across very different plants; for instance, the name "marigold" can refer to Calendula officinalis, which is used to heal skin, or Tagetes, which is often used as an insect repellent but is not typically recognized for medicinal use on the skin. By using scientific names, we ensure that we are speaking of the same plant with the same properties, which is crucial for effective and safe herbal practice.

Herbal actions describe what a herb does in terms of its thera-peutic effects. For example, adaptogens are herbs that help the body resist stressors of all kinds, physical, chemical, or biological, like Rhodiola or ashwagandha, which improve the body's ability to handle stress and fend off fatigue. Antiseptics, like thyme or tea tree, combat infections by inhibiting the growth of bacteria, making them invalu-able in your natural first aid kit. Astringents, such as witch hazel, cause contraction and shrink tissues, which can help tone your skin or stop bleeding. Understanding these actions allows you to choose the right herb for the right situation, much like selecting the appropriate tool for a job.

Lastly, let's briefly outline various methods of preparing herbs, setting the stage for more detailed explorations later in this book. In addition to the tinctures, decoctions, infusions, and salves already discussed, there are also powders, capsules, and syrups, each serving different needs and preferences. Powders are dried plants ground into a fine dust, which can be used in capsules for ease of consump-tion or added to smoothies or food. Syrups, which involve simmering herbs in water with sugar or honey, create a sweet and often soothing remedy that is especially friendly for children or those averse to bitter tastes. Each method has its place, and understanding when and how to use them can enhance the efficacy of your herbal practice.

The Herbalist's Toolkit: Essential Supplies for Homemade Remedies

Embarking on the path of making your own herbal remedies is both exciting and a bit like becoming a kitchen scientist. You don't need a lot of fancy equipment to get started, but having the right tools can make the process more efficient and enjoyable.

Let's begin with the basics. At the very least, you'll need some jars and bottles for storing whatever you make—glass is best because it doesn't react with herbs or essential oils. Dark glass is even better as it helps to protect the contents from light, which can degrade the active compounds in your remedies.

A good quality scale is vital for accuracy, especially when you are following recipes that require precise measurements or when making remedies that will be ingested. It's important to ensure that your measurements are exact to avoid creating something too strong or too dilute, which could affect the efficacy of your final product. Strainers are also necessary; fine mesh strainers or cheesecloth can be used to remove solids from tinctures and infusions, ensuring the texture and clarity of your final product is perfect.

For those who feel more adventurous and wish to delve deeper into herbalism, investing in some advanced equipment can expand your capabilities. A still for distillation can be used for creating essential oils and hydrosols (floral waters). These can be used in aromatherapy or as bases for creams and lotions. If you are serious about making your own extracts, a press is an invaluable tool. Herbal presses extract liquids from macerated herbs, which means you can produce clearer, more concentrated tinctures and oils.

Finding high-quality tools and ingredients can be a journey in itself. For basic supplies like jars, scales, and strainers, kitchen supply stores or online marketplaces are excellent resources. When it comes to more specialized equipment like stills and presses, you may want to look at suppliers who cater specifically to herbalists or the aromatherapy community. These suppliers often provide products that are tailored to the unique needs of herbal remedy preparation.

The importance of sustainability and ethical sourcing in herbalism cannot be overstressed. As herbalists, we have a responsibility to our environment and communities to source tools and ingredients thoughtfully. This means choosing suppliers who are committed to sustainable practices and who source their herbs ethically. It's not just about the quality of the product, but also about supporting a supply chain that respects the earth and its inhabitants. When possible, choose tools that are durable and made from sustainable materials. Opt for herbs that are organically grown and ethically harvested. Sometimes, this might mean choosing locally grown herbs, which can also have the added benefit of supporting local economies and reducing carbon footprints.

As you gather these tools and begin to experiment with making your own remedies, remember that each jar of salve, each bottle of tincture reflects a tradition that spans centuries. These practices connect us to the natural world and to the countless generations who have turned to the earth for healing. Each remedy you craft is a step towards greater self-sufficiency and a deeper connection to the healing powers of nature. Whether you are mixing a simple calming tea or distilling an intricate essential oil, these acts carry deep meaning and tradition, a practice that is both ancient and perpetually new.

Identifying Quality Herbs: Sourcing and Selection

When you begin using herbal remedies, one of the fundamental skills you'll need to develop is identifying and selecting high-quality herbs. While ensuring effectiveness, this ability promotes safety, potency, and allows us to get the most out of our herbal investments. Quality in herbs can be discerned through several indicators such as color, aroma, and texture. Let's dive into how you can become adept at spotting the best quality herbs for your needs.

Color is often the first indication of an herb's quality. Freshness and proper drying and storage processes preserve the vibrant colors of herbs. For instance, high-quality dried peppermint leaves should retain a lively green hue, rather than turning a dull, brownish-green. This vibrancy suggests the presence of active phytochemicals, which are crucial for the herb's therapeutic effects. Similarly, the bright yellow of turmeric root powder is a good indicator of its freshness and curcumin content, its primary active ingredient.

Aroma is another powerful clue. Herbs should have a distinct, clean, and crisp scent that is characteristic of their species. Lavender, for example, should have a rich floral aroma, and any hint of mustiness can indicate mold or improper storage. Texture, too, speaks volumes about an herb's quality. Herbs should feel appropriate to their type: leaves should be crisp and crumble under pressure if dry, roots should be firm and not overly shriveled, and powders should be fine and free from clumps.

Now, understanding your sourcing options can significantly affect the quality of the herbs you use. Growing your own herbs is often seen as the gold standard for ensuring quality because it allows you complete control over the growing conditions, harvest time, and storage practices. This option lets you harvest your herbs at their peak potency and dry them promptly and properly. However, not everyone has the space or time for home gardening, and some climates aren't suitable for growing certain herbs.

Wildcrafting, or gathering herbs from their natural habitat, is another method that can yield potent herbs directly from the earth. This practice connects you deeply with the cycle of the plants and can be a very fulfilling experience. However, it requires a good knowledge of the plants to avoid picking endangered species or those that have been exposed to pollutants. It's crucial to harvest responsibly to ensure sustainability and to avoid damaging the natural habitats.

This leaves us with purchasing from reputable suppliers, which is the most accessible option for many. When choosing this route, you'll want to look for suppliers who provide detailed information about the origin, growing conditions, and harvesting methods of their herbs. Suppliers who can offer organic certification or similar credentials are often a safer bet as this indicates adherence to certain standards in cultivation and handling.

Speaking of organic certification, let's discuss its importance. Organic herbs are grown without synthetic pesticides, herbicides, or fertilizers, and are often handled more carefully throughout the harvesting and drying processes. The absence of these chemicals not only supports your health but also benefits the environment by reducing pollution and enhancing biodiversity. Organic certification isn't always essential for every herb, but it is particularly important for those plants that are prone to heavy pesticide use when grown conventionally, such as chamomile or peppermint. Additionally, if you are consuming herbs specifically for health benefits, opting for organic can prevent the introduction of unwanted chemicals into your body, which might undermine the very health benefits you are seeking to gain.

Lastly, proper storage is critical in maintaining the quality of herbs once they have been harvested or purchased. Always store herbs in a cool, dark place away from direct sunlight, heat, and moisture. Glass containers with airtight lids are ideal for storage as they don't interact with the herbs and prevent contamination. When assessing the quality of packaged herbs, check for any signs of moisture, which can lead to mold, or any discoloration, which might indicate degradation. The packaging should be secure and possibly UV-resistant if the herbs are likely to be exposed to light.

By understanding and applying these principles of sourcing and selecting high-quality herbs, you can significantly enhance the effectiveness and safety of your herbal remedies. Remember, the quality of your herbs is directly linked to the quality of your health outcomes, making it imperative to choose wisely and judiciously. Use these insights to gather the best possible ingredients for your herbal preparations, ensuring that each remedy is as potent and beneficial as it can be.

Recognizing Contraindications and Interactions

When embracing the healing powers of herbal medicine, it's crucial to navigate this path with both enthusiasm and caution. Understanding contraindications, which are specific situations where an herb should not be used because it may cause harm, is foundational to safe herbal practice. For instance, while St. John's Wort is celebrated for its ability to alleviate depression, it can also interfere dramatically with the effectiveness of prescription drugs, including birth control pills and medications for HIV and cancer. This makes it imperative to understand not just the benefits but also the potential risks associated with each herb.

The world of herbal medicine is dotted with nuances, where the interplay between herbs and pharmaceutical drugs can either lead to healing or be a potential for risk. Common interactions include blood-thinning herbs like Ginkgo biloba, which can dangerously enhance the effects of pharmaceutical blood thinners, leading to an increased risk of bleeding. Similarly, herbs such as licorice root, which is beneficial for issues like stomach ulcers and heartburn, can cause potassium levels to fall if taken in large amounts or for an extended period, especially if you're on heart medication. These examples underscore the importance of not just knowing the herbs but understanding how they interact with other substances. This knowledge is crucial in preventing adverse effects and ensuring that the healing potential of herbs is fully realized without compromise.

Addressing the needs of vulnerable populations such as pregnant individuals, children, and those with specific health conditions further highlights the need for a cautious approach. Pregnancy, for instance, necessitates a heightened sense of care as certain herbs can affect hormonal balance or even stimulate uterine contractions, posing risks to the mother or fetus. For example, despite its popularity in natural health circles, the use of blue cohosh for inducing labor is risky and can lead to complications. Children also require smaller doses and herbs that are milder and non-toxic, as their bodies are still developing and they can react differently to herbs compared to adults.

Moreover, individuals with chronic conditions like high blood pressure or diabetes need to be particularly mindful of the herbs they incorporate into their regimen. The use of ginseng might exacerbate hypertension in some cases, despite its health benefits like boosting energy levels and enhancing cognitive function. Such scenarios underline the importance of tailoring herbal practices to individual health profiles to ensure safety and efficacy.

In light of these complexities, the role of professional guidance cannot be overstated. Consulting with healthcare professionals, particularly those knowledgeable in both conventional and herbal medicine, is invaluable before beginning any new herbal regimen. This collaborative approach helps in identifying potential risks and in integrating herbal remedies safely with any existing treatments. It ensures that your journey towards health and wellness through herbs is supported by comprehensive knowledge and safe practices, respecting the powerful effects herbs can have on the body.

Navigating the world of herbal medicine, therefore, requires a balanced approach where our eagerness to explore natural healing is matched with an informed awareness of the potential risks. Understanding contraindications and interactions, considering the specific needs of vulnerable populations, and seeking professional advice are not just cautious steps but essential practices that safeguard health. As we know, with great power comes great responsibility—in this case, the responsibility to practice herbalism with care and respect for the complex nature of the human body and the potent effects of plants.

Storing Your Herbal Remedies: Maximizing Potency

Proper storage of herbal remedies is good practice and a pivotal part of ensuring that the healing potential of these plants is fully realized when you need them most. Like any other naturally derived substance, herbs and their preparations degrade over time. Their potency is highly influenced by the conditions in which they are kept. Understanding and implementing the best storage techniques therefore becomes crucial to preserving their therapeutic qualities for as long as possible.

The first principle to consider is protecting your herbs from light, air, and moisture. These elements are the main culprits in the degradation of herbal products. Light, particularly direct sunlight, can rapidly diminish the color and strength of herbs due to its ultraviolet (UV) rays causing chemical reactions that deteriorate active compounds. To mitigate this, storing herbal remedies in dark, opaque containers is advisable. If using clear glass, ensure they are kept in dark cabinets or drawers where light exposure is minimal.

Air exposure introduces oxygen, which can oxidize and thus destabilize many herbal compounds, altering their effectiveness and safety. Air-tight containers are your best defense against this risk. They not only keep oxygen out but also ensure that the volatile oils, which are responsible for the therapeutic effects of many herbs, do not evaporate over time. Moisture, on the other hand, can lead to mold and bacteria growth, which spoils the herb and can also pose serious health risks. Ensuring your storage containers are moisture-proof and that your herbs are completely dry before sealing them away will help maintain their integrity.

Beyond these, temperature stability also plays a key role. Fluctuating or high temperatures can hasten the degradation of herbs. A cool, stable environment—generally around 25°C (77°F) or cooler—is ideal for prolonging their lifespan. This makes locations like a basement or a pantry away from heat sources and direct sunlight excellent choices for storing your herbal remedies.

Shelf life is another important consideration and varies depending on the form of the herbal preparation. Dried herbs, for instance, can last up to two years if stored correctly. Tinctures and extracts have a longer shelf life, often up to four to five years, thanks to the preserving power of their alcohol or vinegar bases. Oils and salves may keep for about a year, although this can vary based on the type of oil used and the storage conditions. Water-based preparations like teas and decoctions are much more perishable and should ideally be prepared fresh, though they can be stored in the refrigerator for a couple of days if needed.

Labeling and organizing your herbal remedies efficiently is equally essential. Every container should be clearly labeled with the name of the herb, the date it was stored, and any specific instructions for use. This practice will help to easily identify each remedy, track their shelf life, and ensure that they are used when at their best quality.

For those who have a large collection of herbs, maintaining an inventory can be incredibly helpful. This can include details like where the herb was sourced, the batch number, and any other pertinent information that could affect its use. Organization of your herbal storage area ensures that older stocks are used before newer ones, and that no herb is left forgotten until past its prime. This can be as simple as arranging jars and containers in order of their expiry dates, or categorizing them by their type or purpose, such as digestive aids, herbs for skin care, or remedies for colds and flu.

These storage practices will extend your herbs' shelf life and maximize the therapeutic benefits they can provide. This attention to detail will ensure that the effort you put into selecting and preparing your herbs translates into the maximum healing potential for you and your family.

THREE

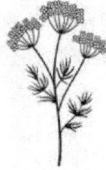

CULTIVATING YOUR HERBAL GARDEN

S tep outside into your own little sanctuary where green leaves flutter gently in the breeze, each one brimming with the potential to heal and nourish. Whether it's a sprawling backyard or a modest balcony space, starting your own herbal garden is a deeply rewarding endeavor that will connect you to the cycle of nature and empower you to take charge of your health. This chapter is designed to guide you through the initial, exciting phase of choosing which herbs to grow, tailored to your environment and needs.

Choosing Your Herbs: Must-Have Plants for Every Beginner

Starting an herbal garden, especially for beginners, can feel like setting out on a great adventure where each choice opens up a world of possibilities. The key to a successful start is selecting the right herbs. These should not only be easy to grow but also versatile in their use, ensuring that your efforts yield tangible rewards right from your doorstep.

One of the first herbs I recommend to new gardeners is basil. This herb is not only straightforward to grow but serves a dual purpose: it's both a culinary star and a medicinal hero. Basil can be sprinkled over a salad to add a fresh, peppery taste, or steeped in hot water to relieve indigestion. Its anti-inflammatory properties make it a practical choice for both your kitchen and your medicine cabinet.

Similarly, mint is another must-have herb. It's incredibly robust, making it perfect for those who are worried they lack a green thumb. From soothing teas that help with digestion to a vibrant addition to dishes, mint is as medicinal as it is culinary. Remember, though, mint tends to spread, so it's often best grown in containers to prevent it from taking over your garden.

When selecting herbs, you will need to consider the specific climate and growing conditions of your area. Lavender, for instance, thrives in hot, sunny, and dry conditions, making it perfect for gardeners in warmer climates. On the other hand, if you live in a cooler, shadier area, you might opt for chives or parsley, which do not require as much direct sunlight and can even prosper indoors. Understanding the climate needs of your herbs will ensure that they grow healthy and potent, ready to be transformed into remedies and culinary delights.

For those who are working with limited space, the art of container gardening becomes invaluable. Herbs like thyme, rosemary, and cilantro can be grown in small pots that fit perfectly on a windowsill or balcony, making them ideal for urban gardeners. Vertical gardening is another innovative solution that maximizes space by using vertical surfaces. Imagine a wall of green, with herbs like creeping rosemary and ivy-leaved nasturtium cascading down. Not only does this make a stunning visual impact, but it also puts fresh herbs right at your fingertips, ready to be plucked and used in your next dish or remedy.

Indoor Herb Gardening 101: Growing Herbs in Small Spaces

Indoor herb gardening is a delightful way to bring a slice of nature into your home, filling your living space with fragrance and greenery while also providing a ready supply of fresh herbs for culinary and medicinal uses. The key to thriving indoor herbs lies in selecting the right containers, understanding light requirements, mastering watering and care techniques, and knowing when to harvest. Let's explore how to create and maintain a vibrant indoor garden.

Choosing the right containers for indoor herb gardening is fundamental. The ideal container should be both functional and fit the aesthetic of your living space. Materials like ceramic, clay, and plastic each have their pros and cons. Ceramic and clay pots are porous, which means they allow air and moisture to move through them, benefiting the roots of the herbs by preventing waterlogging. However, they can be heavy and might require more frequent watering as they allow for quicker soil drying. Plastic containers are lightweight and retain moisture well, which can be beneficial in drier environments but may require careful monitoring to avoid overwatering. Regardless of material, ensure each container has adequate drainage holes to allow excess water to escape, crucial for preventing root rot. Additionally, the size of the container should give your herbs enough room to grow but not so much that the soil stays damp and cold, which can harm the plant.

Light is an important factor to consider when growing indoor herbs. Most common medicinal herbs, such as basil, thyme, and mint, require at least six hours of sunlight a day to thrive. South-facing windows typically provide the most sunlight, but if natural light is limited in your home, growing lights are an effective alternative. These artificial lights mimic the spectrum of sunlight necessary for photosynthesis, and with timers, you can easily regulate the amount of light your herbs receive, mimicking the natural rise and set of the sun. It's a small investment that can significantly boost the growth and health of your indoor garden.

Watering and care are where most new indoor gardeners find challenges, but with a few tips, you can easily keep your herbs healthy. Overwatering is a common issue, as well-watered herbs can quickly become waterlogged if the soil does not drain properly or if the plants are not allowed to dry out between watering sessions. The key is to water deeply but infrequently, allowing the soil to dry out slightly at the top before watering again. This method encourages the roots to grow deeper, searching for moisture and thereby strengthening the plant. Additionally, be mindful of the humidity in your home, especially during winter when indoor air can become quite dry. Herbs like rosemary and thyme thrive in dry conditions, whereas basil and parsley prefer more humidity. Using a spray bottle to mist these plants can help increase humidity levels and replicate their natural environment. Regularly check for pests such as spider mites or aphids, common in indoor settings, and consider natural pest control methods like neem oil or insecticidal soap to keep your garden healthy without the use of harsh chemicals.

Harvesting your herbs effectively is essential to maximize their yield and potency. Regular harvesting encourages growth, so don't hesitate to snip a few leaves for your tea or dinner. Always use sharp scissors or pruning shears to make clean cuts, which help the plant heal faster and continue growing. The best time to harvest most herbs is in the morning after the dew has dried but before the sun is high enough to begin evaporating essential oils, which are at their peak during this time. For continual harvest, never remove more than one-third of the plant at a time. This method ensures that your herbs can recover and continue producing the leaves and flowers that make them so valuable for your kitchen and medicine cabinet.

By understanding and implementing these principles, your indoor herbal garden can flourish, transforming your home into a lush and productive space. Whether it's the simple joy of cooking with herbs you've grown yourself or the satisfaction of preparing a home-made herbal remedy, the benefits of indoor gardening are plentiful and rewarding.

Outdoor Herb Cultivation: Best Practices for Healthy Plants

When choosing the ideal spot for your garden, several factors come into play, all of which will highly impact the well-being of your herbs. Sunlight is perhaps the most important. As mentioned earlier, most herbs such as rosemary, thyme, and basil, thrive in full sun, requiring at least six hours of direct sunlight daily. Therefore, a spot that catches the morning sun could be ideal, as it warms the plants after a cool night, kickstarting their metabolic processes. However, if you reside in a region with extremely hot summers, some afternoon shade will help protect your herbs from being scorched.

Drainage is another critical factor. Herbs generally despise 'wet feet,' meaning they do not like their roots to be waterlogged. An area that slopes slightly is preferable as it facilitates natural water runoff. If your heart is set on a flat area, consider raising your garden beds to improve drainage. Soil quality cannot be overlooked either. Herbs flourish in well-draining soil as it prevents water from pooling around the roots, which can lead to root rot. The ideal soil for most herbs is loamy and enriched with organic matter to provide adequate nutrients. If your garden soil is heavy and clayey, amending it with sand or organic compost can improve its texture and fertility, making it more conducive for herb growth.

Once the perfect site is selected, preparing your soil is your next step. This stage is like setting a strong foundation for a building—it's essential for the long-term health of your garden. Begin by clearing the area of weeds, rocks, and other debris. This cleanup prevents future competition for resources and removes any habitats for pests. Then, test the soil pH since most herbs prefer a neutral to slightly alkaline environment. You can easily adjust the pH by adding lime to increase alkalinity or sulfur to increase acidity, based on the needs of your herbs.

Enriching the soil is next. Mix in well-rotted compost or aged manure into the top 6-8 inches of soil. This organic matter not only improves soil structure and drainage but also slowly releases nutrients into the soil, feeding your herbs throughout the growing season. For an added boost, especially in nutrient-poor soils, a balanced slow-release organic fertilizer can be incorporated at this stage. Remember, healthy soil leads to robust plants, which are more capable of resisting diseases and pests.

Speaking of pests, managing them organically can maintain the health of your garden without resorting to harsh chemicals. Common pests like aphids, slugs, and spider mites can be a nuisance, but nature offers its own solutions. Introducing beneficial insects such as ladybugs and lacewings can help control aphid populations naturally. These predators do not harm the plants but will feast on pests that do. For slugs, barriers made from crushed eggshells or diatomaceous earth can be effective. These materials create a sharp barrier that slugs avoid. Through trial and error, I've also found companion planting highly effective. Growing herbs like garlic and chives can repel certain pests due to their strong scents. Moreover, these plants can enhance the growth and flavor of neighboring herbs, making them invaluable allies in your garden.

Seasonal care is the final piece of the puzzle in maintaining a thriving outdoor herb garden. Each season brings specific challenges and opportunities. In spring, the focus is on planting and early growth. This is a good time to add a layer of mulch around your herbs. Mulch conserves moisture, suppresses weeds, and keeps the soil temperature stable. Summer requires vigilance for pest control and regular watering. Herbs might need additional water during heat waves, but be cautious not to overwater! Autumn is ideal for harvesting and preparing your garden for the colder months. Some perennial herbs like mint and oregano can be divided and replanted to prevent overcrowding and renew vigor. Winter preparation involves protecting your herbs from freezing temperatures. Mulching with straw or leaves can insulate plant roots, and cold frames or cloches can be used for particularly sensitive herbs.

Each of these practices, from thoughtful site selection to seasonal care adjustments, contributes significantly to the vitality of your outdoor herb garden. By creating a natural balance and providing consistent care, you will cultivate a garden of useful herbs within a vibrant ecosystem that supports a wide array of life, enhancing both the beauty and productivity of your space.

Harvesting Your Herbs: Timing and Techniques for Peak Potency

Harvesting your herbs is a delicate dance with nature, timed to capture the essence and strength of your plants at their peak. To optimize the potency of your herbal remedies, understanding the precise moment and method of harvest is crucial. The ideal time to gather your herbs greatly depends on the specific parts of the plant you need and when their key compounds are most concentrated.

For leaves, the best time to harvest is just before the plant flowers, when the energy of the plant is still focused on vegetative growth and the oils are most vibrant. This is when leaves like basil or mint are bursting with aromatic oils, perfect for your culinary dishes or a fresh herbal tea. The optimal time of day for harvesting leaves is in the morning after the dew has evaporated but before the sun is high. This timing ensures that the essential oils, which are volatile and can be diminished by heat, are at their peak concentration.

When it comes to flowers, such as chamomile or lavender, they should be collected when they are fully open and before they begin to fade. This stage ensures that the active constituents are still potent. Like leaves, flowers should be picked in the early morning hours to capture their delicate essences before they are diminished by the day's heat. Roots, on the other hand, are best harvested in the late fall when the plant's energy has returned to the roots for storage over the winter. Dandelion and burdock are prime examples where the roots contain valuable nutrients and should be dug up when the aerial parts of the plant begin to die back.

The techniques used to harvest different parts of the plant are vital for the quality of your herbs and for ensuring the continued health and productivity of your plants. Leaves should be snipped using sharp scissors or pruners to avoid tearing, which can damage the plant and open pathways for disease. When harvesting flowers, it's often best to cut them with a small portion of stem attached, which can help in handling and later processing. Roots require a more hands-on approach; they should be carefully dug out of the ground with a garden fork or spade, taking care not to cut or break the roots in the process. After lifting, shake off excess soil and wash them gently to remove any remaining dirt.

Post-harvest handling is equally important to maintain the herbs' therapeutic properties. Once harvested, leaves and flowers can be used fresh, or they may require drying or other forms of preservation. However, they should first be inspected for pests and any diseased or wilted parts should be removed. Washing should be done sparingly, as water can strip away some of the volatile oils and potent compounds. If washing is necessary, do it gently under a stream of cool water and pat the herbs dry immediately with a soft towel.

To maximize the potency of your herbs, the methods of processing are critical. Drying should be done quickly after harvest to prevent decay and the growth of mold. Herbs can be tied in small bunches and hung upside down in a warm, dry, airy space, away from direct sunlight. This method helps maintain their color and essential oils. For roots, cleaning followed by immediate chopping and drying or processing can help preserve their active ingredients. When handled correctly, these herbal parts can be transformed into powerful extracts, tinctures, or dried ingredients for your apothecary.

Understanding these nuances of harvesting and post-harvest handling allows you to capture the full medicinal potential of your garden. It is a beautiful way to connect with the cycle of growth and renewal in nature, turning the act of harvesting into both a science and an art.

Drying and Preserving Herbs: Ensuring Year-Round Supplies

I often think of the art of drying and preserving herbs similar to capturing and locking away the essence of summer, to be enjoyed throughout the year. This process is a wonderful way to ensure that the vibrant flavors and healing properties of your garden continue to enrich your life, even when your plants have gone dormant. Each method of drying, from air drying to using modern dehydrators, has its unique benefits and suitability depending on the type of herbs you are working with and the resources available to you.

Air drying is perhaps the oldest and most energy-efficient method of preserving herbs. It works best in environments that are warm and dry with good air circulation. To air dry herbs, simply tie them into small bundles and hang them upside down in a warm, airy room. Alternatively, you can lay them out on a screen or a clean, dry surface. This method is particularly effective for herbs with high moisture content, such as mint or basil, as it allows them to dry slowly and naturally, retaining much of their essential oils and flavor. However, it's important to ensure that the area is free from moisture and not exposed to direct sunlight, as these can lead to the degradation of the herbs' potent qualities.

For those seeking a quicker, more consistent method, oven drying can be a viable option. This method involves laying herbs on a baking sheet and allowing them to dry in an oven set at a very low temperature (ideally between 100°F to 110°F). The door of the oven should remain slightly open to allow moisture to escape. This method is faster than air drying and can be particularly useful on humid days when air drying might not be as effective. However, it requires careful monitoring to ensure that the herbs do not burn or lose their volatile oils due to excessive heat.

Over the years, I've found that using a dehydrator offers the most control over temperature and air flow, making it an excellent choice for preserving herbs in optimal condition. Dehydrators are designed to circulate air and maintain a constant temperature, which can be adjusted according to the delicacy of the herbs. This method is ideal for herbs that are particularly sensitive to heat and light, as it preserves their color and essential properties effectively. While dehydrators can be an investment, for avid gardeners and herbalists who regularly preserve large quantities of herbs, the consistency and efficiency they offer can be well worth the cost.

Testing for proper dryness is crucial to prevent mold and decay in stored herbs. Herbs should feel dry and crumbly to the touch, and stems should snap rather than bend. Leaves should crumble easily. Any remaining moisture can lead to mold growth once the herbs are stored, which can render them unusable and potentially harmful. If you're unsure whether your herbs are dry enough, consider placing a small amount in an airtight container for a day. Check the container for any condensation after 24 hours; if moisture is present, further drying is needed.

Once dried, storing your herbs correctly is key to maintaining their quality and potency. Glass jars with airtight lids are ideal for storage as they prevent exposure to air and light, both of which can degrade the quality of the herbs over time. Be sure to label each jar with the name of the herb and the date it was stored. Store these jars in a cool, dark place to further protect them from temperature fluctuations and light. Properly stored, dried herbs can retain flavor and potency for up to a year.

When it comes to using your preserved herbs, understanding how to adjust for potency can enhance their effectiveness in recipes and remedies. Dried herbs are generally more potent than fresh, as the drying process concentrates their flavors and oils. A good rule of thumb is to use one-third the amount of dried herb to fresh when substituting in recipes. For teas or infusions, rehydrating the herbs by steeping them in hot water can release their flavors and medicinal properties effectively. If the aroma or flavor seems diminished, gently crushing the herbs between your fingers before use can help to release any remaining oils, revitalizing their potency.

By mastering these techniques of drying and storing, you will be able to enjoy an abundance of herbal delights to enhance your cooking and healing practices all year round.

Ethical Wildcrafting

Wildcrafting, the practice of gathering plants from their natural, often wild habitat, holds a special allure for those of us who seek a deeper connection with nature. It is an age-old method that taps into the bounty of the earth, allowing us to source herbs directly from the environment where they thrive. This practice is a way to obtain ingredients for culinary and medicinal purposes while offering us the opportunity to interact with the natural world, creating appreciation and respect for the ecosystems that nurture these plants.

It should be noted that wildcrafting must be approached with care and responsibility to ensure that it does not harm the plants or their native habitats. Sustainability is the cornerstone of ethical wildcrafting. It involves understanding and practicing the careful management of plant populations to avoid depleting resources. Sustainable foraging means taking only what you need and no more than what the plant population can afford to lose. It's crucial to familiarize yourself with the growth cycles of the plants you gather. For instance, if a plant is early in its growth cycle and has not yet flowered, taking too much could prevent it from reaching maturity and reproducing. Always leave enough plants behind to ensure that the population can regenerate.

Another aspect of sustainable foraging is the method of harvest. For roots, for instance, it's advisable to take only part of the root system, allowing the plant to continue growing. This method can be applied by carefully digging around the plant, removing part of the root, and then replanting the remaining part with some soil amendments to help it recover. When harvesting leaves, flowers, or seeds, use clean, sharp tools to make precise cuts, which help the plant to heal more quickly and reduce the risk of disease. It's also beneficial to scatter seeds of the plants you harvest (if it's the right season for seeding) to aid in the natural regeneration of the population.

Legal considerations are also paramount when wildcrafting. Many areas have specific laws and regulations regarding the foraging of wild plants to protect endangered species and preserve natural habitats. It's important to research and understand the laws in your region. Some areas may require permits or have restrictions on the amount and type of plants that can be foraged. National parks, for instance, often prohibit the removal of any natural materials to preserve the ecological balance. Always ensure that you have the proper permissions and understand the local guidelines before you start foraging.

Safety and proper identification are equally critical in wildcrafting. Misidentifying plants can have serious consequences, especially when dealing with wild herbs that are used for medicinal purposes. Some plants have toxic look-alikes, and mistakes can lead not only to ineffective remedies but also to harmful or potentially life-threatening reactions. Invest time in learning about the plants in your area. Use reliable field guides, participate in workshops, and consider joining foraging groups where experienced foragers can provide guidance. Always cross-reference multiple sources before picking and using a plant, and when in doubt, it's safer to leave a plant than risk an incorrect identification.

The practice of wildcrafting brings with it a responsibility to both the plant populations and the ecosystems where they exist. By adhering to sustainable practices, respecting legal restrictions, and prioritizing safety and accurate identification, you'll ensure that wildcrafting remains a viable and enriching practice that can continue for generations. This mindful approach will help preserve the natural heritage while deepening your connection with the environment, enhancing your appreciation for the web of life that supports the growth of these medicinal plants.

From the basics of choosing and growing your plants, whether indoors or outdoors, to the ethical considerations of wildcrafting, you are now well-equipped to move forward and transform these plants into remedies and recipes that will enrich your life.

Herbal Journaling

To personalize your herbal gardening journey, take a moment to reflect. List the herbs that you are interested in growing. Next to each, note down why you've chosen them—be it for their health benefits, ease of growth, or culinary uses. Then, research how well they might grow in your local climate and space. This will help you create a tailored garden plan that aligns with your health goals and environmental conditions.

FOUR

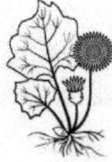

PREPARING HERBAL REMEDIES

> "Plants possess an innate wisdom that can help us unlock our own healing potential."
>
> ALCHEMY OF HERBS

D iving into the world of preparing your own herbal remedies is likely to unlock a new realm of personal empowerment and connection to the natural world. There is so much beauty to be found in transforming the life force of plants into nourishing and healing concoctions that resonate with your body's own rhythms and needs. Here, we'll begin with one of the most ancient and accessible forms of herbal preparations: the art of tea blending.

Therapeutic Herbal Teas for Everyday Wellness

The creation of therapeutic herbal teas is as much an art as it is a science. It starts with understanding the individual properties of herbs and how they can synergistically combine to enhance each other's effects. When blending teas, balance is key—not just in flavor, but also in the therapeutic attributes each herb brings to the cup. For instance, a tea meant to aid digestion might include peppermint for its soothing properties and fennel for its ability to relieve gas and bloating. The goal is to create a blend where the herbs work together harmoniously to address specific health concerns while providing a pleasing flavor profile.

Each herb holds a spectrum of flavors—from the deep earthiness of dandelion root to the light floral notes of chamomile. The challenge and beauty of tea blending lie in achieving a balance that pleases the palate and supports health. It's important to start with small batches, experimenting with different ratios, until you find the blend that meets your taste and therapeutic needs. This process involves so much more than following recipes; it is about engaging your senses and intuition, allowing you to connect deeply with the ingredients and their origins.

Common Recipes

LET'S explore some specific recipes that target common health concerns. For a soothing bedtime tea, a blend of chamomile, lavender, and valerian root works wonders. Chamomile calms the nervous system, lavender contributes a relaxing aroma, and valerian root acts as a natural sleep inducer. To aid digestion, a mix of peppermint, ginger, and a touch of licorice can be effective. Peppermint relieves stomach discomfort, ginger stimulates digestion, and licorice can soothe inflammation in the digestive tract.

For those dealing with stress, a tea combining lemon balm, rose petals, and ashwagandha can help restore a sense of calm and balance. Lemon balm is known for its ability to ease anxiety and promote relaxation, rose petals add a floral lift that can soothe the heart, and ashwagandha is an adaptogen that helps the body cope with stress.

Brewing Techniques

To MAXIMIZE the medicinal properties of herbal teas, proper brewing techniques are essential. Unlike brewing regular tea, most herbal teas benefit from a longer steeping time to fully extract their benefits. A general rule is to steep for at least 10-15 minutes, covered, to prevent the escape of aromatic oils and other volatile substances. Some roots and barks may require a longer steeping time or even a gentle simmer to release their active compounds.

Water temperature is also crucial and varies depending on the delicacy of the herbs used. While robust herbs like ginger and hawthorn can withstand boiling water, more delicate herbs such as lavender and rose petals are better steeped in water just off the boil to preserve their subtle flavors and therapeutic oils.

Storage and Freshness

To PRESERVE the flavor and medicinal qualities of herbal teas, proper storage is key. Dried herbal blends should be stored in airtight containers away from direct sunlight and heat, which can degrade their potency over time. Glass jars with airtight seals are ideal as they protect the herbs from moisture and light. Label each container with the date of blending; most herbal teas can maintain their potency for up to a year if stored correctly.

Maintaining the freshness of your teas not only involves good storage practices but also starts with the quality of the herbs you use. Sourcing high-quality, organic herbs, and storing them properly before blending will ensure that each cup of tea is as potent and beneficial as possible.

Tea Tasting Diary

To deepen your understanding and enjoyment of herbal teas, jot down your impressions when trying new blends. You may want to include flavors, aromas, and the effects you notice on your well-being.

Crafting Tinctures and Elixirs

The crafting of tinctures and elixirs represents a fascinating aspect of herbal medicine, harnessing the potent properties of plants in concentrated forms. These liquid extracts offer a practical and effective way for you to incorporate the benefits of herbs into your daily routine. Let's explore the meticulous process of creating tinctures, which involves macerating (soaking) herbs in alcohol to extract their active compounds.

The first step in tincture preparation is selecting your herb. Whether it's the calming properties of lavender or the immune-boosting power of echinacea, the choice of herb depends on the effects you are seeking. Once you have your dried herb, the next step is maceration. Here, precision in proportion is crucial—typically, a ratio of one part herb to four parts alcohol is used, but this can vary depending on the herb's density and water content. Begin by finely chopping or grinding your herb to increase the surface area, which allows the alcohol to extract compounds more effectively.

Place the herb in a clean, dry jar, and cover it with a high-proof alcohol, such as vodka or brandy, which acts as a solvent to draw out the soluble active compounds. The alcohol also acts as a preservative, allowing your tincture to maintain its potency over long periods. Seal the jar tightly and store it in a cool, dark place, shaking it daily to mix the contents. This process is typically maintained for about four to six weeks to allow thorough extraction.

After the waiting period, the next phase is straining. Line a funnel with cheesecloth and place it over a second clean jar. Pour the tincture through the funnel, allowing the liquid to filter through and leaving the solid herb parts behind. Squeeze the cheesecloth to extract as much liquid as possible. Your tincture is now ready to be transferred into smaller dropper bottles for easy use. Label each bottle with the herb name, date, and any specific instructions for use, such as dosage or dilution.

Transitioning to elixirs, these delightful concoctions are essentially tinctures sweetened with natural ingredients like honey, glycerin, or maple syrup, making them more palatable, especially for those who might find the strong alcohol base of tinctures too harsh. Elixirs not only improve the flavor but can also enhance the medicinal properties of the blend, as many sweeteners have their own health benefits. For example, honey is known for its antibacterial properties and can soothe inflammation, making it an excellent addition to a throat-soothing tincture of marshmallow root and licorice.

To craft an elixir, begin with a prepared tincture. Decide on a suitable sweetener and consider any additional flavors or herbal extracts that might complement the base tincture. For a simple elixir, a ratio of one part sweetener to three parts tincture can be used as a starting point. Combine the ingredients in a clean bottle, shake well to mix, and taste. Adjust the sweetness or add more herbs according to your preference. As with any herbal preparation, creativity plays a crucial role. You might experiment with adding citrus peels for a zesty flavor or vanilla beans for a warming, comforting note.

Considering dosages for tinctures and elixirs, it's important to start with small amounts and observe how your body responds. A general guideline is to begin with 1-2 milliliters of tincture, taken 2-3 times per day, although this can vary widely depending on the herb's strength and the individual's needs. For elixirs, because of their added sweetness, a starting dose might be a teaspoon (approximately 5 milliliters), also taken 2-3 times per day. Always consult with a healthcare provider or a knowledgeable herbalist to determine the best dosage for your specific health circumstances, especially if you are managing a health condition or are pregnant or breastfeeding.

The creation of tinctures and elixirs is a wonderful way to engage deeply with the properties of plants, blending science, art, and intuition. As you explore the vast possibilities in combining herbs, embrace the learning process, and allow your understanding and appreciation of herbal medicine to grow. Perhaps, like myself, you will find that these potent liquid extracts offer much convenience and efficacy, while empowering you to take control of your health in a most natural way.

Herbal Salves and Balms: Natural Solutions for Skin Care

Creating herbal salves and balms is a deeply rewarding process that combines the healing properties of herbs with the protective qualities of waxes and oils. These topical preparations are wonderful for treating a variety of skin issues, from everyday dryness to more acute conditions like cuts and bruises. The foundation of any good salve or balm lies in understanding the roles of its components: the infused oils that carry the medicinal properties of herbs, the beeswax that solidifies the mixture, and any additional elements like butters or essential oils that enhance the product's skin-soothing properties.

The first step in making a salve or balm is the infusion of herbs into a carrier oil. Commonly used oils include olive, coconut, or almond oil, chosen for their own beneficial skin properties. The herbs you choose depend on the desired effect of the salve. For instance, calendula is renowned for its soothing and regenerative properties, making it ideal for healing salves, whereas arnica is excellent for balms aimed at bruise and pain relief. To infuse, herbs are typically steeped in oil over low heat for several hours, ensuring that the active compounds are extracted into the oil. This herbal oil is then strained and serves as the base for the salve or balm.

Beeswax plays a crucial role as it not only thickens the oil to create a spreadable balm but also acts as a protective barrier on the skin, sealing in the herbal benefits and moisture without clogging pores. The general rule of thumb for salve making is to use approximately one part beeswax to four or five parts infused oil, depending on the desired consistency. For balms, which are typically firmer, a greater proportion of beeswax might be used. The oil and beeswax are gently heated together until the wax melts, at which point any additional ingredients such as shea butter or vitamin E oil can be added for extra nourishing properties.

Formulating recipes for specific skin conditions involves selecting herbs that target those issues. For dry and cracked skin, a salve made from a blend of chamomile and marshmallow root infused in sweet almond oil, with added cocoa butter, can be particularly healing. Chamomile soothes irritation while marshmallow root provides a mucilaginous property that hydrates and softens the skin. For a balm that aids in the healing of cuts and bruises, combining comfrey and plantain infused in olive oil, with added tea tree oil for its antimicrobial properties, makes an effective remedy. Comfrey promotes cell regeneration, speeding up the healing process, while plantain works as an anti-inflammatory.

Packaging and storage of salves and balms are important to maintain their efficacy. Once the salve or balm has been poured into containers—typically small jars or metal tins—and cooled, they should be labeled clearly with ingredients and the date of manufacture. Natural products like these generally have a shelf life of up to one year, provided they are stored in a cool, dark place. Exposure to heat can cause the salve to melt and potentially spoil, as the oils can go rancid.

When applying herbal salves and balms, a little goes a long way. They should be massaged gently into the skin, allowing the warmth of your skin to melt the balm and increase absorption. It's important to ensure the area of application is clean to avoid trapping any dirt or bacteria under the protective layer of the balm. Regular use can significantly improve skin conditions and also serve as a soothing ritual, connecting you to the natural ingredients and their origins.

Through the process of crafting your own herbal salves and balms, you will gain both a useful product and an intimate knowledge of the ingredients and their benefits. This knowledge can be incredibly empowering in helping you to take control of your skin care, customizing products that cater specifically to your body's needs.

Each batch of salve or balm reflects the healing power of nature and our own ability to harness it.

Herbal Capsules: Creating Your Own Supplements

The convenience and precision of herbal capsules make them a favored choice for many who seek to include herbs in their daily health regimen. Capsules allow you to consume herbs in a form that is easy to take while bypassing the often earthy and bitter tastes of some medicinal plants. This can be particularly appealing if you are incorporating herbs like turmeric or valerian, known for their strong flavors, into your wellness practices. Let's explore the transformative process of turning dried herbs into your very own custom capsules.

Creating capsules begins with the proper preparation of the herb, which involves drying and grinding the plant material into a fine powder. This step is crucial as it increases the surface area of the herb, allowing for better extraction of the active compounds when consumed. To start, ensure that your chosen herbs are completely dry. Any moisture can cause the powder to clump and can lead to spoilage when stored. Once dried, the herbs are ground using a coffee grinder or a specialized herb grinder. This process should be done gradually, checking frequently to achieve a fine consistency without overheating the herbs, which could lead to a loss of potent volatile oils.

The texture of the final powder is paramount; it should be fine enough to pack tightly into capsules but not so fine that it becomes airborne easily. If you find the powder too coarse, it can be sifted through a fine mesh to separate larger bits, which can be re-ground. The goal is a homogenous powder that will ensure each capsule contains an equal distribution of the herb's therapeutic properties.

Next, the filling process can be approached manually or with the help of a capsule-filling machine, which can be particularly useful when making large batches or when precision is imperative for thera-peutic reasons. If filling capsules by hand, you will need empty capsules, which come in different sizes according to the dose required. Start by separating the top and bottom of the capsules. Using a small spoon or a capsule machine's spreading card, gently pack the powdered herb into the longer part of the capsule, ensuring it is tightly filled. Once filled, rejoin the top and bottom halves of the capsules. This method, while more labor-intensive, can be seen as an opportunity for a meditative engagement with the herbs.

For those who prefer efficiency or need to produce larger quantities, capsule-filling machines are invaluable. These devices allow you to fill multiple capsules simultaneously and often include a tamper to compact the herb powder firmly. The process involves spreading the powder over a tray of capsule bottoms, tamping down the powder, and then capping them with the tops. This method ensures consistency in dosage and is significantly faster than manual filling, making it ideal for those who rely on herbal supplements for daily health management.

Storage and labeling of herbal capsules are as important as their preparation. Proper storage ensures the longevity and efficacy of the capsules. Once filled, the capsules should be stored in airtight containers to protect them from moisture and light, which could degrade the active compounds. Glass jars with tight-sealing lids are perfect for this purpose. It's advisable to store them in a cool, dry place to prevent any potential degradation from heat. Each container should be labeled clearly with the name of the herb, the date of capsule production, and the expiration date, which is generally one year from making if stored correctly.

Remember that labeling should also include dosage recommendations, which can vary depending on the potency of the herb and the individual's needs. These recommendations should be based on thorough research or consultations with a healthcare provider knowledgeable in herbal medicine. This attention to detail helps in maintaining an organized system and ensures safety and effectiveness in the use of your herbal capsules.

By embracing the process of making your own herbal capsules, you will be able to gain control over what you consume while deepening your understanding of the herbs and their benefits. Whether you are managing a chronic condition, seeking to enhance your overall wellness, or simply exploring the rich world of herbal medicine, creating your own capsules is a great way to tailor your health supplements to your specific needs, ensuring that you receive optimal therapeutic benefits.

Syrups and Tonics: Sweet Remedies for Coughs and Energy

The crafting of herbal syrups and tonics is a delightful tradition that marries the robust benefits of herbs with the comforting sweetness of natural sugars. These preparations show the versatility and adaptability of herbal remedies, providing both soothing comfort for ailments like coughs and colds, and a vital boost of energy when needed. The process of making these remedies involves a careful simmering of chosen herbs in water to extract their beneficial properties, followed by the addition of a sweetening agent to create a pleasant, often delicious, liquid remedy.

When you set out to make a herbal syrup, your choice of herbs should be guided by their known benefits for treating specific conditions. For example, to create a syrup particularly effective for coughs, herbs such as marshmallow root, which provides a soothing mucilage, and thyme, which serves as a powerful antimicrobial agent, can be used. The roots or leaves are gently simmered in water until the essence of the herbs is extracted into a potent decoction. This usually takes about 20-30 minutes of simmering after which the liquid is strained to remove the plant matter, ensuring a smooth final syrup.

Once you have your herbal decoction, it's time to transform it into a syrup by adding a sweetener. This not only improves the flavor but also increases the syrup's preservative properties. Honey is a popular choice due to its soothing effects and antibacterial properties, making it ideal for cough syrups. However, if you're preparing remedies that might be used by individuals who prefer vegan options, or for children under one year where honey is not recommended, alternatives like maple syrup or vegetable glycerin can be used. These sweeteners still provide an excellent consistency and sweetness, with glycerin adding a slightly smooth texture that's pleasant in a throat syrup.

Enhancing the flavor and therapeutic potential of your syrups and tonics can be creatively achieved with the addition of natural ingredients like lemon, ginger, or cinnamon. Lemon adds a refreshing zest and vitamin C, boosting the immune-enhancing properties of your syrup. Ginger offers a warming effect, which can be comforting in remedies for colds, and its anti-inflammatory properties make it an excellent choice for soothing sore throats. Cinnamon not only brings a delightful spice but also has antibacterial and antiviral properties that can enhance the syrup's effectiveness against cold symptoms.

Again, preservation is crucial in extending the shelf life of your homemade syrups and tonics. While sugar and honey naturally help preserve these liquid remedies, additional steps can ensure their longevity and maintain their therapeutic qualities. Storing your syrups in sterilized, airtight glass bottles helps prevent contamination and preserve the contents effectively. Refrigeration is also recommended, as it significantly slows down the degradation process. Most homemade syrups can be kept for up to a month when refrigerated. For an added layer of preservation, especially for syrups that may not be used quickly, adding a small amount of alcohol, such as brandy or vodka, can extend the shelf life. This method is particularly useful for tonics meant to be used as health boosters rather than for immediate illness relief, as the alcohol acts as a potent preservative, allowing you to store the tonic for several months under proper conditions.

You will certainly find that each batch you brew has much to offer, including relief and vigor. Whether soothing a sore throat with a marshmallow root and honey syrup or boosting your energy with a ginseng and maple tonic, the remedies you create are sure to offer comfort and vitality, embodying the sweet side of herbal medicine.

Infusions and Decoctions

When you delve into the practice of making herbal infusions and decoctions, you are engaging in one of the most traditional methods of extracting the potent benefits from plants. Both techniques are steeped in history and are fundamental to harnessing the therapeutic properties of herbs, yet they serve different purposes and are used under different circumstances. Understanding when and how to use each method can greatly enhance the effectiveness of the remedies you create.

As we've already seen, an infusion is typically used with the more delicate parts of the plant—leaves, flowers, and sometimes fine stems. This method involves pouring boiling water over the plant parts and letting them steep for a period, usually between 10 to 30 minutes, which extracts the herbs' active compounds. Think of it as making tea, which is, in fact, a common form of infusion. Decoctions are used for the tougher parts, like roots, bark, and seeds. Here, the plant materials are actually simmered in boiling water for a longer duration, typically from 20 minutes to several hours. This process breaks down the plant's cell walls and releases the soluble active compounds into the water.

Let's walk through the process of preparing a standard infusion. Begin by boiling your water. Once it reaches a rolling boil, pour it over about one to two teaspoons of dried herbs for every cup of water in your heat-proof container. Covering the container is crucial as it traps the steam and helps to keep the volatile oils from escaping, which are often responsible for both the aroma and the medicinal properties. After about 15 to 20 minutes, strain the mixture to separate the liquid from the plant parts. The result is a potent, aromatic herbal infusion that can be enjoyed immediately or stored for later use.

Decoctions require a bit more time and attention. Start with cold water and your chosen dried herbal materials, using about one tablespoon of herbs for each cup of water. Place these in a saucepan, and slowly bring the mixture to a boil. Reduce heat and simmer, covered, for about 20 to 45 minutes. The length of simmering time can be adjusted depending on the herb and how strong you want the decoction to be. After cooking, strain the liquid from the herbs. Decoctions are typically stronger than infusions and are often used when the therapeutic goal requires deeper extraction, such as when dealing with tough roots or dense seeds.

The therapeutic uses of infusions and decoctions are varied and rich. A simple peppermint leaf infusion can relieve symptoms of indigestion and soothe an upset stomach, while a decoction of burdock root might be used to cleanse the blood or improve skin health due to its deeper, more potent extraction methods. Echinacea, commonly used to boost the immune system, can be prepared as an infusion to help ward off colds or as a decoction to treat an ongoing respiratory infection.

When it comes to storing these preparations, it's important to note that while potent, they do not have the long shelf life of tinctures or dried herbs. Freshly prepared infusions can be stored in the refrigerator for up to 24 hours. After this, the potency begins to diminish, and the risk of microbial growth increases. Decoctions can be kept a bit longer, typically up to 48 hours under refrigeration. Always store them in airtight containers to minimize exposure to air and light, which can degrade their quality. When consuming, both infusions and decoctions can be enjoyed warm or cold, depending on the nature of the remedy and personal preference. Some find that gently reheating the decoction, not boiling, can make it more palatable and soothing, especially when dealing with cold or flu symptoms.

This exploration into the art of making infusions and decoctions opens up a world of possibilities for using herbs in their most natural and potent forms. As you experiment with these techniques, you'll gain a hands-on understanding of how different parts of the plant can be utilized to support holistic health. Whether you're soothing a sore throat with a slippery elm bark decoction or calming your nerves with a lavender flower infusion, the knowledge you gain from these practices will empower you to take control of your health in the most natural way possible.

We've now journeyed through various methods from tea blending to crafting tinctures, and mastering infusions and decoctions. The next chapter will build on these foundations, guiding you through the integration of herbal remedies into daily life, ensuring that these ancient practices translate into modern wellness solutions.

FIVE

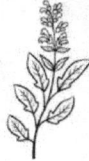

BIOHACKING THE IMMUNE SYSTEM

Your body is not unlike a mighty medieval castle—stone walls, a mighty drawbridge, maybe even a fire-breathing dragon for extra flair. And standing guard? Your immune system, a squad of tireless warriors fending off invaders like stress, germs, and whatever was lurking on that grocery cart handle you *totally* meant to sanitize.

But here's the thing: even the strongest fortresses need reinforcements. In today's world of sleepless nights, processed foods, and enough stress to make a monk twitch, your immune system could use some backup. Luckily, nature has your back. This chapter is all about the plant-powered allies that help fortify your defenses, keep you thriving, and make sure you're ready to take on whatever life throws your way.

Key Herbs for Immune Support

In the vast array of herbs that grace our earth, a few stand out for their potent immune-boosting properties. Echinacea, elderberry, and astragalus – to name a few – are powerful allies in our quest for health. Echinacea is often the first line of defense at the onset of cold symptoms, prized for its ability to kickstart our immune response. Elderberry follows closely, with studies showing its efficacy in reducing the duration and severity of colds, thanks to its high levels of antioxidants and vitamins. Astragalus, a staple in traditional Chinese medicine, is revered for its deep immune-modulating effects, often used to enhance vitality and fight off chronic infections.

Mechanisms of Action

THE SECRET TO THESE HERBS' effectiveness lies in their complex biochemical makeup, which supports the immune system through various pathways. Echinacea, for example, contains compounds like alkamides, which enhance phagocytosis, an immune response in which cells engulf harmful invaders. Elderberry's flavonoids, such as quercetin, are powerful antioxidants that protect cellular health and have antiviral properties. Astragalus boosts the immune system by increasing the production of white blood cells, which are crucial for fighting off pathogens.

Research Backing

THE EFFICACY of these herbal aids is not just anecdotal; numerous studies support their benefits. For instance, research published in the "Journal of International Medical Research" found that Echinacea effectively reduces the symptoms and duration of common colds when taken at the first sign of symptoms. Similarly, a study in the "Journal of Functional Foods" highlights how elderberry substantially reduces upper respiratory symptoms. Such studies not only reinforce the traditional use of these herbs but also help us understand their role in modern medical practices.

Holistic Benefits

BEYOND THEIR DIRECT IMMUNE-BOOSTING EFFECTS, these herbs offer holistic benefits that contribute to overall well-being. The anti-inflammatory properties of Echinacea can alleviate skin conditions and improve skin health, while the antioxidants in elderberry play a crucial role in heart health and may reduce the risk of chronic diseases. Astragalus, with its adaptogenic properties, helps the body cope with stress, enhancing overall energy and vitality. Thus, incorporating these herbs into your daily regimen can lead to broad-spectrum health improvements, reinforcing your body's resilience.

Health Diary

To PERSONALIZE your approach to boosting your immune system, start by noting any frequent illnesses like colds or feelings of fatigue. As you incorporate immune-supporting herbs into your routine, keep a record of any changes in your health. This practice will help you recognize patterns over time and empower you to make informed decisions about your health, based on direct personal observations.

Preparing Immune-Boosting Herbal Blends

Creating blends of herbs that synergistically enhance immune function is an art. Blending herbs is rooted in understanding the unique characteristics each herb brings to the table and how these characteristics can complement each other to fortify your body's defenses. Let's explore how you can craft your own immune-boosting herbal concoctions, tailored to your personal needs and preferences, ensuring you're as protected as possible against common pathogens.

The principle of synergy in herbal blends implies that the combined effect of the herbs can be greater than the sum of their individual effects. To achieve this synergy, start by selecting herbs that support the immune system in different ways. For instance, combining an herb that acts as an immune stimulant, such as garlic, with herbs that provide nutritional support, like nettle, which is rich in vitamins, creates a blend that both stimulates the immune response and nourishes the body. Additionally, adding adaptogens like Siberian ginseng can help enhance the body's overall resilience to stress, which is often a precursor to immune dysfunction.

When crafting recipes for herbal blends, it's important to consider both the therapeutic intent and the flavor profile. For a basic immune-supporting tea, you might start with echinacea, known for its infection-fighting properties. To this base, add elderflower, which has antiviral effects and a pleasantly sweet flavor, complementing the somewhat pungent taste of echinacea. For a touch of warmth and to boost circulation, which helps the immune cells move more efficiently through the body, consider adding ginger. This will bring a spicy kick to the tea and offer anti-inflammatory benefits. To prepare this tea, use about one teaspoon of each herb per cup of boiling water, steeping for about 15 minutes to ensure the active ingredients are well extracted.

Tinctures are another effective way to utilize immune-boosting herbs, as they offer a more concentrated and often more shelf-stable option. A tincture combining astragalus, goldenseal, and licorice root can be particularly potent. Astragalus serves as a deep immune tonic, supporting the increase of white blood cells, while goldenseal has strong antibacterial properties, and licorice root acts as a soothing agent, which also has antiviral benefits. The process involves macerating the herbs in a mixture of alcohol and water, typically at a ratio of 1:5 (herb to menstruum), and letting this sit for about a month, shaking daily. After straining, the tincture can be taken in small doses, such as 1-2 ml, up to three times a day during the immune-compromising seasons or situations.

Personalization of these recipes is key to making them a part of your daily routine. Consider the flavors and forms of administration you prefer, and adjust the recipes accordingly. If you find the taste of tinctures too strong, they can be diluted in a little water or mixed into a beverage like tea or juice. If you are particularly sensitive to certain herbs, adjust the ratios or substitute with other herbs that have similar properties but are better tolerated by your body.

Safety is paramount when dealing with herbal remedies, especially considering dosage and potential interactions with other medications. It's important to start with lower doses of new herbal blends to monitor how your body responds. Gradually increasing the dose as needed can help avoid any adverse reactions. Consultation with a healthcare provider is advisable, particularly if you have underlying health conditions or are taking prescription medications, as some herbs can interact with medications, altering their effectiveness or leading to side effects. For instance, herbs like goldenseal should not be taken with certain over-the-counter drugs and prescription medications as they can interfere with their metabolism.

Whether sipping on a carefully crafted herbal tea or integrating a custom tincture into your wellness routine, the benefits of these natural preparations can be profound and lasting, providing you with the tools you need to support your body's defenses through every season.

Herbs and Nutrition: Foods that Support Herbal Immune Boosters

When it comes to our health, the interplay between herbs and nutrition can have a significant impact. By integrating immune-boosting herbs with nutrient-rich foods, we're concocting a powerful recipe for robust immunity. Let's explore how to seamlessly blend these natural allies into our daily meals, enhancing their collective strength to fortify the body's defenses.

Among the pantheon of foods that complement immune-strengthening herbs, vitamin C-rich fruits and zinc-containing seeds stand out for their pivotal roles. Vitamin C is a powerful booster for your immune system, a critical antioxidant that helps protect your body's cells from damage. Fruits like oranges, kiwis, and strawberries not only make a delightful pairing with immune-enhancing herbs like echinacea but also increase the bioavailability of herb-derived compounds through their acidic content, which aids in nutrient absorption. On the other hand, seeds such as pumpkin and sesame are laden with zinc, a mineral essential for immune function. Zinc acts by supporting the normal development and function of cells mediating innate immunity, which includes cells that can destroy bacteria and infected host cells. When these seeds are incorporated into meals with astragalus, an herb known for its profound immune-boosting properties, they help in creating a fortified barrier against pathogens.

Integrating these powerful foods and herbs into your daily meals requires a mindful approach that doesn't just focus on the individual qualities of these components but also on how their combinations can enhance your overall well-being. Start by considering the meals you enjoy and how they can serve as vehicles for these immune-supporting elements. For breakfast, a smoothie might be the perfect option. Blend berries high in vitamin C with a spoonful of elderberry syrup, which offers antiviral properties, and a dash of powdered astragalus to fortify your immune system right from the start of your day. For lunch or dinner, think of incorporating garlic and onions, natural immune boosters due to their powerful antibacterial and antiviral properties, into soups or stews. Add turmeric, with its potent anti-inflammatory benefits, and black pepper, which increases the absorption of turmeric's active compound, curcumin, to boost the dish's health-promoting properties.

Recipe Ideas

To BRING this integration to life, let's dive into a specific recipe that marries these concepts deliciously. Imagine a warm quinoa salad— quinoa, a complete protein providing all nine essential amino acids, tossed with roasted pumpkin seeds for zinc, and pomegranate seeds for a burst of vitamin C. Dress this mixture with a vinaigrette made from olive oil, lemon juice, and a generous drizzle of honeyed ginger syrup, a concoction that not only adds a zesty sweetness but also brings the anti-inflammatory and immune-boosting properties of ginger. This dish not only satisfies the palate but also turns each bite into an immune-boosting delight.

As you make these dietary enhancements, consider the broader lifestyle changes that might amplify the benefits of your herb and nutrition-focused diet. Regular physical activity, adequate hydration, and sufficient sleep are foundational to immune health. Pairing these lifestyle habits with your dietary practices creates a holistic approach to immunity. Engage in moderate exercise to improve blood circulation, which helps the immune system function more efficiently. Ensure you're drinking plenty of fluids throughout the day to help flush toxins from your body and maintain the health of your lymphatic system, a crucial component of your immune system. Prioritize sleep, aiming for 7-9 hours per night, as sleep has a direct impact on immune function and the effectiveness of the healing properties of herbs and nutrients in your diet.

By embracing these nutritional allies and incorporating them thoughtfully into your meals, you significantly bolster your body's natural defenses. This proactive approach to health, where every meal is an opportunity to nourish and protect your body, is not just about prevention but also about empowering you to take control of your health through the everyday choices you make. I urge you to continue to explore and integrate these powerful natural resources into your life, keeping in mind that each step you take is a step toward a healthier, more vibrant you, supported by the best of what nature has to offer.

Seasonal Immune Support: Tailoring Your Approach

As the world around us changes with the seasons, so too does the need of our immune system. It is a dynamic entity, sensitive to the shifting environments and distinct challenges each season presents. Understanding the seasonal variations in immune system require-ments can help you adjust your herbal support accordingly, ensuring your body remains resilient year-round. In the colder months, your immune system can be severely tested; the chilly weather forces us indoors where viruses can thrive and the lack of sunlight reduces our natural vitamin D levels, an essential component for immune defense. Conversely, the summer brings its own set of challenges, including increased exposure to allergens and the need to maintain hydration to support immune function.

During winter, the focus is often on preventing and fighting the common cold and flu. This is where herbs like Andrographis come into play. Known in traditional medicine as the "King of Bitters," Andrographis paniculata has been shown in numerous studies to significantly enhance the immune response, reducing the severity and duration of cold and flu symptoms. Integrating this herb into your daily regimen as winter approaches can be an effective way to bolster your defenses. Another invaluable ally for the winter months is the Reishi mushroom. Revered in Asian cultures for its immune-modulating effects, Reishi can be taken in the form of a tea or supplement to help maintain immune fortitude during this taxing season.

As the world blossoms in spring and the heat intensifies in summer, the challenges for your immune system shift predominantly towards combating allergies and maintaining hydration. Stinging nettle is a powerhouse for spring and summer. Acting as a natural antihistamine, it helps alleviate allergic reactions by blocking the body's ability to produce histamine. It can be consumed as a tea or in capsule form to help manage seasonal allergies effectively. Additionally, herbs like peppermint provide a cooling effect during the hot months and promote respiratory health by relaxing the muscles of the respiratory tract. This makes it easier to breathe when allergens are high and the air is heavy with pollen.

To optimize your immune health throughout the year, incorporating preventative strategies into your daily life can be incredibly beneficial. One effective practice is rotating your herbal supplements seasonally. Just as you might change your wardrobe to suit the weather, adapting your herbal regimen can help address the changing needs of your body. Start by introducing immune-strengthening herbs as teas or tinctures a few weeks before the season changes. This proactive approach can help prepare your body for the upcoming environmental shifts and challenges. For instance, beginning your intake of Andrographis or Elderberry a few weeks before winter can prime your immune system to ward off common viral infections typically prevalent during the cold months.

In addition to herbal preparations, maintaining a lifestyle that supports immune health is crucial. Regular physical activity, which can vary in intensity with the seasons, helps boost circulation and general health, thereby supporting the immune system. In summer, activities might include swimming or early morning jogs to avoid the midday heat, while in winter, indoor yoga or pilates classes can keep you active even when it's cold outside. Ensuring adequate sleep is a cornerstone of good immune health; it's when you sleep that your body repairs itself and regenerates. Make sure to adjust your sleeping environment according to the seasonal needs—cool and airy in the summer, warm and cozy in the winter—to promote restful sleep.

By tuning into the needs of your body and adjusting your herbal support and lifestyle according to the seasons, you will create a dynamic health practice that anticipates the needs of your immune system and enhances your overall well-being. This seasonal approach to immune health is also about nurturing a state of mind & body wellness that is dynamic, capable of adapting to the ever-changing world around us.

Herbal Vaccines: Myth Busting and Facts

In the realm of herbal medicine, the term "herbal vaccines" often surfaces, wrapped in a mix of hope and misconception. Within the context of this book, I think it important to address these myths head-on and to clarify the scientific facts, ensuring you can make informed decisions about your health. Understanding the distinction between traditional vaccines and what is often termed as "herbal vaccines" is essential.

Traditional vaccines are biologically prepared antigens that can generate an immune response to protect against specific bacteria or viruses. On the other hand, "herbal vaccines" is a term that can be misleading as no herbal remedies can induce an immune response akin to what's achieved with conventional vaccines.

Of course, many herbs do significantly bolster the immune system's ability to fight infections and disease, but they do not work in the same way as vaccines. For instance, herbs like garlic and oregano exhibit strong antimicrobial properties that can help the body ward off and fight infections. However, they do not teach the immune system to recognize and combat future attacks of the same pathogens, which is the primary function of a vaccine. Clarifying this distinction helps in understanding the role that herbs can play in overall immune health without expecting them to replace the critical function of clinical immunizations.

Discussing the supporting role of herbs in relation to conventional vaccines, it's important to note that some herbs have been identified to potentially enhance vaccine efficacy. For instance, studies have shown that herbs like echinacea can support the immune system's general function, potentially aiding in a stronger response to vaccines. However, it's crucial to consult healthcare professionals before combining herbal supplements with vaccinations, as the interaction between herbs and the vaccine components may vary.

In terms of supporting science, there are numerous studies that highlight the immune-modulating properties of certain herbs which can complement the effects of vaccines. For example, research has shown that astragalus can enhance the body's immune response by increasing the production of white blood cells, which play a crucial role in fighting infections. This does not imply that astragalus acts as a vaccine, but it does suggest that in conjunction with vaccinations, it might help the body mount a better immune response.

For those interested in exploring this intersection of herbalism and immunization further, there are several resources that can provide reliable information. Academic journals such as the Journal of Ethnopharmacology often publish studies on the effects of medicinal plants on the immune system. Websites maintained by professional herbal organizations like the American Botanical Council offer articles, research summaries, and links to studies concerning herbal medicine and immune health. These platforms provide valuable insights that can help you understand both the capabilities and the limits of herbal remedies in the context of immune health.

Navigating the world of herbal remedies and vaccines requires access to accurate, evidence-based information. By debunking myths and understanding the actual benefits and functions of herbal treatments, you can make informed decisions that effectively enhance your health and well-being. Moreover, engaging with professional resources ensures that your approach to using herbs in supporting your immune system is both safe and effective, grounded in scientific research rather than mere conjecture.

Managing Autoimmune Conditions

Navigating the complexities of autoimmune conditions, where the body's immune system mistakenly attacks its own tissues, requires a nuanced understanding of immune system function and the factors that influence its behavior. Autoimmune diseases, such as rheumatoid arthritis, lupus, and multiple sclerosis, pose unique challenges due to their chronic nature and the unpredictable episodes of flare-ups and remission. These conditions can profoundly impact quality of life, making effective management strategies essential.

Among the holistic tools available, certain herbs have shown promise in modulating the immune system's responses, potentially easing the inflammation and pain associated with autoimmune disorders. Turmeric, with its active compound curcumin, stands out for its potent anti-inflammatory properties. Extensive research has shown that curcumin can inhibit molecules that play a significant role in inflammation, which is a central feature of autoimmune diseases. Ginger, another herb renowned for its medicinal properties, contains gingerol, a bioactive substance with powerful anti-inflammatory and antioxidant effects. Regular inclusion of ginger in your diet or as a supplement could help manage symptoms by reducing systemic inflammation and enhancing overall wellness.

However, while these herbs offer potential benefits, the approach to using them in the context of autoimmune conditions must be highly individualized. Autoimmune diseases vary greatly in their manifestation and impact from person to person; what works for one individual may not be effective for another. This variability underscores the importance of customization in herbal therapy. It involves careful consideration of the specific autoimmune condition, the individual's unique physiological responses, and any concurrent treatments they might be undergoing. For instance, while turmeric is generally beneficial, it can exacerbate symptoms in people with certain conditions such as gallbladder disease. Hence, understanding the nuances of each herb and its interactions with your body is crucial.

Consultation with healthcare providers is an indispensable part of this process. Before integrating any new herbal remedy into your routine, especially if you are managing an autoimmune condition, discussing it with your doctor or a qualified herbalist is essential. They can provide guidance based on your medical history and current treatments, helping to avoid any potential adverse reactions or interactions with prescribed medications. For example, herbs like turmeric might interact with blood-thinning medications, increasing the risk of bleeding, a critical detail that requires medical oversight.

Integrating herbs into the management of autoimmune conditions also involves considering how they can complement conventional treatments. Many patients find that a combination of pharmaceutical treatments for managing acute flare-ups and herbal remedies for long-term symptom control works best. This integrative strategy not only addresses the symptoms more comprehensively but also focuses on enhancing overall well-being, which is often compromised in autoimmune diseases. For instance, adopting an anti-inflammatory diet rich in omega-3 fatty acids, antioxidants, and phytonutrients, alongside targeted herbal supplements like turmeric and ginger, can create a supportive health regimen that minimizes the impact of the disease on daily life.

This careful, personalized approach to using herbal remedies offers a pathway to better managing the complexities of autoimmune conditions, enhancing quality of life, and promoting long-term health. It emphasizes the importance of understanding the underlying mechanisms of action of these herbs, the necessity for individual customization, and the value of professional guidance. By considering these factors, you can safely and effectively incorporate herbal remedies into your overall strategy for managing autoimmune conditions, taking proactive steps towards a balanced and healthier life.

Diving into the next chapter, we will shift our focus to alleviating stress and anxiety, where you will learn how herbal remedies can restore balance and peace to your hectic life, complementing the robust immune support strategies we've developed here.

SIX

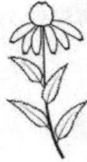

BIOHACKING STRESS AND ANXIETY

I f modern life had a theme song, it would be the sound of twenty-five unread emails, a buzzing phone, and the *ding* of yet another calendar reminder. Stress and anxiety? Oh, they're practically on your VIP guest list, showing up uninvited, overstaying their welcome, and raiding your mental snack cabinet.

But here's the good news: nature has been dealing with stress way longer than we have. Long before group chats and back-to-back meetings, ancient healers turned to plants—calming chamomile, soothing lavender, grounding ashwagandha—to quiet the noise and restore balance. This chapter is your invitation to do the same. Think of it as a deep breath in book form, a place where each page offers a moment of calm, a sip of herbal wisdom, and a reminder that you *can* reclaim your peace.

Understanding Stress: How Herbs Can Help

Stress, at its core, is the body's response to perceived threats or demands, a complex orchestration of hormonal and physiological reactions that prepare us to fight or flee. When you encounter stress, your body releases a flood of hormones including adrenaline and cortisol, which heighten your heart rate, increase your blood pressure, and boost energy supplies. While this response is vital for survival, its chronic activation in daily modern life can lead to debilitating effects on both mental and physical health. The nervous system, particularly the autonomic system, plays a crucial role here, maintaining an involuntary control over the heart, lungs, and other organs that are directly impacted during stress episodes.

Herbal Soothers: Nature's Antidote to Stress

HERBS LIKE LAVENDER, Chamomile, and Ashwagandha are like gentle warriors. Each offers a unique set of calming properties that help soothe the storm of stress within. Lavender, with its sweet floral scent, is a delight to the senses and a profound relaxant, known to ease tension and promote a peaceful state of mind. Chamomile, often sipped in teas before bedtime, serves as a mild tranquilizer, its delicate blossoms working to soothe nerves and alleviate anxiety. Ashwagandha, a revered herb in Ayurvedic medicine, acts as an adaptogen, meaning it helps your body manage stress more effectively, reducing cortisol levels and enhancing your resilience to stressors.

The Science Behind the Soothing

THE EFFICACY of these herbs lies in their bioactive compounds that interact with your body in a way that mitigates stress. Lavender contains linalool, a terpene alcohol, which has been shown to reduce anxiety by affecting the brain through its calming aroma and direct interactions with GABAergic systems, which regulate nerve excitability. Chamomile is rich in apigenin, a flavonoid that binds to benzodiazepine receptors in the brain, offering a sedative effect without the side effects of pharmaceutical relaxants. Ashwagandha, on the other hand, works by moderating the hypothalamic-pituitary-adrenal (HPA) axis, thereby regulating the stress response and fostering a sense of balance.

Complementary Practices: Enhancing Herbal Effects

WHILE HERBS ARE powerful on their own, their stress-relieving effects can be significantly amplified when combined with practices like yoga and meditation. Yoga, with its emphasis on breath control and physical postures, complements the physiological benefits of herbs by reducing muscle tension and lowering blood pressure, enhancing the overall calmness. Meditation, particularly mindfulness meditation, trains your mind to focus on the present moment, reducing the chaotic thoughts that often fuel anxiety and stress. Integrating these practices into your routine can create a holistic approach to managing stress, where herbs provide the biochemical support and yoga and meditation contribute to a balanced mental state.

Top Herbs for Anxiety and Stress Relief

In the quest to find tranquility in the hustle and bustle of everyday life, certain herbs offer natural ways to alleviate anxiety and stress. Among these, St. John's Wort, Kava Kava, and Lemon Balm stand out for their effectiveness, as well as for the depth of research backing their use. These herbs have been used traditionally across different cultures, and today they are appreciated for their roles in modern herbal therapy. Understanding the specific benefits and applications of each can guide you to make informed choices about incorporating these herbal allies into your life.

St. John's Wort, scientifically known as Hypericum perforatum, is renowned for its ability to treat mild to moderate depression and anxiety. Its active ingredients, hypericin and hyperforin, are thought to influence neurotransmitter activity in the brain, enhancing mood and providing a calming effect. For those dealing with anxiety, the standard dosage often recommended is 300 mg of St. John's Wort extract three times a day, standardized to 0.3% hypericin content. This herb can be taken in the form of capsules or as a tea. However, one should brew the tea with care, steeping it for about ten minutes to allow the active compounds to release into the water without degrading them.

Kava Kava, or Piper methysticum, is another herb known for its potent anti-anxiety properties. It originates from the Pacific Islands, where it has been used for centuries in ceremonial drinks to induce a sense of relaxation and well-being. The active compounds in Kava, known as kavalactones, work by modulating GABA receptors in the brain, similar to how certain anti-anxiety medications operate. It is typically consumed as a beverage or taken in capsule form, with a common dosage ranging from 100 to 250 mg of kavalactones per day. Preparing a traditional Kava drink involves steeping the root powder in water and then straining it to produce a mild, earthy tea that offers a noticeable sense of relaxation shortly after consumption.

Lemon Balm, or Melissa officinalis, is an herb in the mint family with a gentle lemon scent and is highly valued for its soothing effects on the nervous system. This herb helps to reduce anxiety and promote sleep by increasing GABA levels in the brain, thus decreasing excitability and fostering a state of calm. Lemon Balm can be enjoyed as a fresh tea, using about 1 to 2 teaspoons of dried leaves steeped in hot water for up to ten minutes. This method extracts the herb's essential oils and active compounds effectively, making for a soothing, aromatic drink that eases the mind and lifts the spirits.

Incorporating these herbs into your daily routine can be a comforting ritual that alleviates stress and enhances your overall sense of well-being. As usual, it's important to consider the safety aspects and potential interactions of these herbs, especially if you are currently taking pharmaceutical medications. St. John's Wort, for instance, is known to interact with a variety of medications including antidepressants and birth control pills, potentially diminishing their effectiveness. Kava Kava, while effective, has been linked to liver toxicity in rare cases, particularly when used in large doses or for prolonged periods. It is crucial to source these herbs from reputable suppliers and to consult with a healthcare provider before starting any new herbal regimen, particularly if you have existing health conditions or are on other medications.

The personal testimonials of individuals who have found relief through these herbs can be both inspiring and informative. For instance, case studies recounting the experiences of long-term anxiety sufferers who have successfully integrated Lemon Balm into their daily routines, describe not only reduced anxiety levels but also improved sleep and overall vitality. These stories show the potential of herbal remedies to significantly enhance quality of life when used appropriately and with respect for their potent nature.

Always keep in mind that what works wonderfully for one individual might not be as effective for another. Patience and persistence, paired with a mindful approach to understanding and using these herbal remedies, are key to integrating them successfully into your stress management practices.

Herbal Baths and Soaks for Relaxation

Immersing yourself in the warm, fragrant waters of an herbal bath can be likened to stepping into a serene oasis, where the stresses of the day dissolve as easily as the herbs infuse their essence into the water. Crafting this tranquil experience within the confines of your bathroom is simpler than it may seem, and it begins with selecting the right herbs that cater not only to relaxation but also to your personal scent preferences and skin needs.

Herbs such as rose petals, known for their soothing aroma and skin-softening properties, or eucalyptus, recognized for its clear, invigorating scent and respiratory benefits, are excellent starters. To prepare your bath, you'll want to either bundle loose herbs in a muslin cloth or use a large tea bag, allowing the active compounds to disperse without leaving residue that could clog your drain.

The process of setting up your herbal bath should be as calming as the bath itself. Begin by filling your tub with warm water, adjusting the temperature to your comfort. As the tub fills, hang your bag of herbs directly under the faucet, letting the water run through them, which helps release their essential oils and fragrances effectively. This method ensures a more potent herbal infusion. For a truly immersive experience, consider the timing of your bath. Allowing the herbs to steep in the bath as it fills and letting the concoction sit for a few minutes before you enter can significantly enhance the potency of the herbal benefits, making your soak not just about cleanliness but a therapeutic ritual.

Creating specific recipes for your relaxation needs adds a personalized touch to your herbal baths. For a soothing, stress-relieving soak, a blend of lavender, chamomile, and valerian root works wonders for calming both the mind and the body. Lavender and chamomile are renowned for their gentle sedative properties, while valerian root amplifies this effect, making it ideal for pre-sleep bathing rituals. Alternatively, for a more uplifting experience, combining citrus peels, such as orange or grapefruit, with mint leaves can invigorate the senses and rejuvenate the spirit. These blends cater beautifully to different emotional needs while offering a variety of aromatic delights, ensuring that your bath is as pleasing to the nose as it is soothing to the skin and soul.

To elevate your bathing experience further, incorporating elements like essential oils and ambient music can transform your bathroom into a spa-like environment. A few drops of essential oils like sandalwood or jasmine can be added directly to the bathwater or mixed with the herbs for deeper aroma infusion. These oils enhance the natural fragrances of the herbs and offer additional therapeutic benefits, such as improved mood and decreased anxiety. Complement this with soft, soothing background music or nature sounds, which can help in reducing stress levels and enhancing the overall relaxation effect. This combination of herbal benefits, aromatic indulgence, and auditory bliss creates a multisensory experience that can help alleviate not just physical tension but also mental and emotional stress.

Incorporating herbal baths into your regular self-care routine is an excellent choice for sustained stress management and overall well-being. Setting aside specific days of the week or moments in your day for this practice can help establish a rhythm that your body and mind will instinctively begin to recognize and respond to. Over time, this routine becomes a signal to your system, indicating that it's time to unwind and let go of the day's stresses. It's not just about the act of bathing but about creating a consistent practice that your body and mind come to anticipate and rely on for relaxation and rejuvenation. This regularity will also contribute to long-term stress management and an overall more balanced, relaxed state of being.

Aromatherapy: Essential Oils for Emotional Well-being

In the world of natural health, aromatherapy emerges as a graceful and potent ally, wielding the essence of botanicals to harmonize the mind and alleviate the strains of anxiety and stress. This practice, which harnesses the aromatic compounds of plants known as essential oils, offers a direct pathway to emotional balance through the olfactory system. When you inhale these fragrant molecules, they interact with the limbic system, the brain's area responsible for emotions, memory, and arousal. This interaction can trigger changes in mood and mental state, making aromatherapy a powerful tool in managing daily tensions and anxieties.

Let's explore the foundational elements of aromatherapy, beginning with how it can be seamlessly integrated into your life to foster tranquility and reduce stress. Essential oils, the potent liquids extracted from flowers, leaves, bark, and roots, contain the essence of the plant's therapeutic properties. When diffused into the air or applied to the skin, these oils can have a calming, uplifting, or balancing effect, depending on their specific properties. For instance, consider the soothing influence of rose oil, which can alleviate stress and promote a sense of peace, or the invigorating effect of peppermint oil, which can energize the mind and dispel feelings of irritability or fatigue.

The safety of using essential oils is paramount, as their concentrated nature means they can be potent. It is crucial to dilute them properly before topical application to avoid skin irritation. A general guideline for safe dilution is to use about 6 drops of essential oil per ounce of carrier oil, such as jojoba or sweet almond oil. Additionally, certain oils like bergamot and other citrus oils can make the skin more sensitive to sunlight, known as photosensitivity, and should be used with caution if you're planning to be outdoors.

Diverse techniques exist for applying essential oils, each serving different needs and preferences. Diffusers are popular and certainly one of my favorite methods. They have the ability to disperse a fine mist of oil-infused water into the air, creating an ambiance that can elevate mood and reduce stress. Alternatively, topical application, enhanced through the use of carrier oils, allows the oils to be absorbed through the skin, providing more localized benefits. Techniques such as the hand-inhalation method, where a few drops of oil are rubbed between the palms and inhaled deeply, offer a quick and effective way to harness the benefits of essential oils, especially on-the-go.

Creating your own blends of essential oils can be a deeply rewarding experience, allowing you to customize scents and therapeutic properties to suit your specific emotional and physical needs. For beginners, starting with a simple combination that targets stress relief can be particularly beneficial. A basic yet effective recipe might include lavender, known for its relaxing properties; frankincense, which is grounding and mood-enhancing; and sweet orange, which adds a bright, uplifting note to the blend. To create this blend, combine 5 parts lavender, 3 parts frankincense, and 2 parts sweet orange. Adjust the ratios based on your scent preferences and the desired therapeutic effect. This blend can be used in a diffuser or diluted with a carrier oil for massage or topical application.

With aromatherapy, each inhalation can be considered an opportunity to imbibe the healing essence of the earth, a moment of connection between you and the natural world. You will certainly find that adding this practice to your stress management toolkit will offer a delightful and effective way to enhance your emotional well-being through the power of nature's fragrances.

Creating a Calming Herbal Routine

Establishing a routine that incorporates herbal remedies can be a transformative practice that not only manages stress and anxiety but also enhances overall well-being. Imagine starting your day not with the harsh blare of an alarm, but with the soothing aroma of herbal tea steaming gently beside your bed. Envision closing each evening with a ritual that unwinds the mind and prepares the body for restorative sleep. It is possible to craft such routines, tailored to integrate seamlessly with your lifestyle and personal preferences, ensuring it becomes a sustaining rather than taxing part of your life.

Daily Routines

To EFFECTIVELY MANAGE stress and anxiety, consider how herbal remedies can be included in your daily schedule. It can begin with understanding the natural rhythm of your day and identifying moments that typically invite stress or when you feel its effects most acutely. For many of us, mornings can be rushed and tense, making them ideal for integrating calming herbal supplements. Consider a capsule of Rhodiola rosea, an adaptogen known for enhancing mental performance and reducing fatigue, taken with breakfast to set a grounded tone for the day. Throughout the day, keep a bottle of lemon balm hydrosol at your desk; a quick spritz around your workspace not only refreshes the air but also offers a moment of mental clarity and stress relief.

As the day winds down, transition to herbs that support relaxation and prepare your body for sleep. A cup of passionflower tea after dinner can be excellent for this purpose. Known for its mild sedative properties, passionflower helps soothe the mind from the day's worries and eases the transition into the night's rest.

Morning Rituals

MORNINGS SET the tone for the day, and starting them in a state of calm can profoundly impact your stress levels and general outlook. Establishing a morning ritual around calming herbal teas or supplements can be a delightful way to awaken your senses and prepare mentally for the day ahead. A warm cup of tulsi tea, also known as holy basil, makes for an excellent start. Revered in Ayurveda for its stress-reducing properties, tulsi helps modulate cortisol levels, keeping stress under control from the morning onward. If tea is too time-consuming, a green tea extract supplement can also invigorate the body while providing theanine, an amino acid that promotes relaxation without drowsiness.

Evening Wind-Down

THE IMPORTANCE of effectively winding down at the end of the day cannot be overstated, especially in our fast-paced world. Creating an evening ritual that includes herbal elements can significantly enhance the quality of your sleep, a crucial factor in stress management and overall health. A relaxing herbal routine might include a warm bath infused with lavender essential oil, known for its soothing properties, followed by a cup of chamomile tea, which has been used for centuries to reduce inflammation, alleviate pain, and induce sleep. For those who find the ritual of preparing tea soothing, this can be a meditative practice in itself, helping to signal to your body that the day is ending and it's time to slow down.

Personalizing Your Herbal Routine

THE KEY to sustaining any routine is ensuring it aligns with your personal needs and lifestyle. Adaptability is crucial; what works for one person might not work for another, and your own needs may change over time. Listen to your body and be willing to adjust your herbal practices as required. For instance, if you find that chamomile tea is too mild, you might switch to valerian root, known for its stronger sedative properties. If morning teas are too cumbersome, encapsulated supplements might provide a more convenient alternative. The goal is to make the use of herbal remedies is a flexible, enjoyable part of your life, not another source of stress.

Meditation and Herbs: A Synergistic Approach to Stress

In the quest for tranquility within the whirlwind of daily responsibilities, the pairing of meditation and herbal remedies can be a profoundly effective alliance. This combination not only deepens the relaxation experienced during meditation but also enhances the overall resilience against stress. Integrating herbs such as Gotu Kola and Holy Basil into your meditation practice can elevate the experience by promoting greater mental clarity and peace.

Meditation, in its essence, is a practice of focus and mindfulness, a method to quiet the mind and cultivate a state of calm observance. When complemented with herbal aids, particularly those that enhance cognitive function and soothe the nervous system, the effects can be markedly enhanced. Gotu Kola, for instance, is renowned not just for its ability to improve circulation but also for its impact on cognitive functions. It supports memory and neural pathways, making it an excellent herb to incorporate before a meditation session focused on clarity and mindfulness. Similarly, Holy Basil, or Tulsi, acts as an adaptogen, helping the body cope with stress and supporting inner calm. When consumed as a tea prior to meditation, it prepares the mind and body to enter a more profound state of relaxation, making the session more effective.

The technique of integrating these herbs into meditation can vary based on personal preference and the specific effects desired. One effective method is to prepare a tea infused with either Gotu Kola or Holy Basil about thirty minutes before beginning your meditation. This timing allows the body to assimilate the herbs' benefits, aligning your peak state of calm with your meditation practice. Alternatively, creating an ambient space with diffused essential oils, such as those derived from these herbs, can also enhance the sensory experience, facilitating a deeper meditative state.

The many stories I have heard from individuals who have combined these practices highlight significant improvements in their ability to manage stress and anxiety. For example, a dear friend of mine – a woman in her forties - integrated Gotu Kola into her morning meditation routine. Previously overwhelmed by the pace of her high-stress job, she found that this combination progressively enhanced her focus throughout the day and instilled a sense of serenity that she carried into her work interactions, which dramatically improved her overall quality of life.

SEVEN

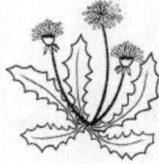

BIOHACKING GUT HEALTH

Your body is a complex ecosystem where every microorganism plays a critical role. Just as a symphony falls apart without harmony among its instruments, so does our health without the balanced interaction of the billions of bacteria living in our gut. In this chapter, we will look into the fascinating world of the gut microbiome, revealing how these microscopic inhabitants profoundly influence our overall health—from the robustness of our immune system to the state of our mental well-being. We'll explore how simple, natural remedies like herbs can play a pivotal role in nurturing this fundamental aspect of our health.

The Gut-Health Connection

The gut microbiome, a complex community of bacteria, fungi, and viruses, resides predominantly in our intestines and has a monumental task: it influences our digestion, immune function, and even our emotions and mental health. Each person's microbiome is as unique as their fingerprint, shaped by factors such as diet, lifestyle, and genetics. Scientists and doctors now recognize that a healthy microbiome is not just about digestion – it is also essential for synthesizing certain vitamins, processing waste, and forming a barrier against harmful bacteria and infections. Remarkably, it also communicates with the brain through what you may know as the gut-brain axis, which impacts our mood, stress levels, and even behaviors.

Herbs for Gut Health

IN THE WORLD of natural health, certain herbs have been celebrated for their powerful effects on digestive health. Peppermint, for instance, is a spasmolytic, which means it can relieve spasms in the gut and reduce the discomfort from irritable bowel syndrome (IBS). Ginger, with its potent anti-inflammatory properties, has the potential to ease nausea while also playing a role in protecting and healing the gut lining. Slippery Elm, rich in mucilage, acts as a demulcent, soothing the mucous membranes of the gut and promoting healing from within. These herbs, among others, offer gentle yet effective ways to support gut health and ensure the microbiome is thriving.

The actions of these herbs on the digestive system are both gentle and profound. Peppermint relaxes the smooth muscles of the digestive tract, easing the passage of food and reducing symptoms of bloating and gas. Ginger stimulates digestion through its warming effects, encouraging the body to break down food more efficiently and absorb nutrients effectively. Slippery Elm forms a protective layer on the lining of the digestive tract, helping to calm inflammation and repair damage, which is particularly beneficial for those with conditions like gastritis or ulcerative colitis. Integrating these herbs into your daily regimen can significantly enhance gut function and contribute to a more balanced microbiome.

Lifestyle Factors

I WOULD LIKE to take a moment here to mention the importance of recognizing that while herbs offer substantial benefits, they are part of a broader lifestyle approach to gut health. Factors like diet, stress, sleep, and exercise all play integral roles. Of course, all of these factors can be enhanced by the support of appropriate herbal remedies – there's a win-win situation!

A diet rich in diverse, fiber-rich foods feeds the good bacteria in the gut, promoting diversity and resilience. Also, managing stress through practices like yoga and mindfulness can reduce inflammation and gut disturbances, often exacerbated by a hectic lifestyle. Of course, adequate sleep and regular physical activity also contribute to a healthier microbiome, enhancing gut motility and immunity.

Natural and Herbal Remedies for Gut Health

Ginger

- Reduces nausea
- Enhances digestion
- Anti-inflammatory

Use in cooking, take as supplements, or add fresh ginger to smoothies or tea.

Peppermint

- Soothes stomach pain
- Reduces bloating
- Supports bile flow
- Relieves IBS symptoms

Drink peppermint tea or use peppermint oil capsules.

Turmeric

- Reduces inflammation
- Supports digestion
- Promotes gut flora

Add to curries, soups, or take as supplements or use in smoothies or golden milk.

Fennel

- Relieves bloating
- Supports digestion
- Balances gut flora

Use in cooking, chew fennel seeds or drink fennel tea.

Aloe Vera

- Soothes digestive tract
- Supports gut healing
- Reduces inflammation
- Aids in detoxification
- Relieves burn and skin irritation pain
- Accelerates skin healing

Use in smoothies, apply topically or drink aloe vera juice.

Licorice Root

- Eases stomach pain
- Heals gut lining
- Reduces inflammation
- Supports digestion

Drink licorice root tea, consume liquorice capsules or chewable tablets, or mix with aloe vera to reduce skin inflammation.

Chamomile

- Reduces inflammation
- Soothes gut lining
- Reduces indigestion

Use in herbal infusions, Use to create soaps, scrubs, and skin care products, in a soothing bath, or simply infuse for a calming cup of tea.

Integration Tips

A FEW GENTLE REMINDERS....

- **Daily Routine**: Incorporate herbal teas like ginger, peppermint, and chamomile into your daily routine.
- **Meals**: Use gut-friendly herbs like turmeric and fennel in cooking.
- **Supplements**: Consider herbal supplements for concentrated benefits.
- **Hydration**: Ensure you drink plenty of water throughout the day, including herbal infusions.
- **Exercise**: Move your body in ways that allow it to feel alive! Practice physical activities and movement that cater to your personal needs and abilities.
- **Mindfulness**: Practice stress management techniques such as meditation or yoga to support overall gut health.

AS YOU BEGIN to practice these natural solutions and lifestyle adjustments, you will find that the benefits extend farther than improved digestion. All of these will immensely contribute to enhancing your immune system, stabilizing your moods, and potentially transforming your overall health.

Herbs for Digestive Support

In the gentle unfolding of natural wellness, the role of herbs in supporting our digestive health is quite essential. Each herb possesses a unique signature of support, from stimulating a sluggish appetite to easing the discomfort of bloating. Understanding the nuanced benefits of these herbal allies can transform our approach to digestive health, offering tailored solutions that resonate with your body's needs.

Among the many herbs dedicated to digestive support, Fennel, Caraway, and Artichoke leaf stand out. Fennel, with its sweet, licorice-like taste, has long been cherished for its ability to alleviate gas and bloating. Its seeds contain anethole, a compound that relaxes the smooth muscles of the digestive tract, facilitating the release of trapped gas and easing abdominal discomfort. Caraway seeds, on the other hand, are known for their carminative properties that not only help in expelling gas but also improve digestion by promoting the growth of healthy gut flora. Artichoke leaf extract is celebrated for its ability to stimulate bile production, which is essential for fat digestion and vitamin absorption, making it particularly beneficial for those experiencing sluggish digestion.

The preparation of these herbs is as important as their selection. To harness the benefits of Fennel and Caraway, a simple tea can be made by steeping the seeds in hot water for 5 to 10 minutes. This method allows the essential oils and active compounds to infuse into the water, creating a soothing, warm beverage that can be enjoyed after meals to aid digestion.

Artichoke leaf, however, is best consumed as an extract or tincture to capture its full range of digestive benefits. Integrating these into meals can also be delightful; fennel seeds can be added to breads or chewed directly after a meal, and caraway seeds make a flavorful addition to cheeses and salads, enhancing the dish while providing digestive support.

The personalization of herbal treatments is also key in addressing individual digestive challenges. Not everyone will have the same reaction to an herb, and what works for one person might not work for another. This is where the art of herbal customization comes into play. For instance, if you find that your digestion is particularly sensitive to high-fiber foods, incorporating soothing herbs like Marshmallow root, which forms a protective gel over the digestive tract, can be beneficial. Conversely, if you are prone to indigestion, bitter herbs like Gentian root can stimulate digestive enzymes and improve food breakdown and nutrient absorption.

As mentioned previously, integrating these herbs into a holistic dietary approach enhances their effectiveness. Combining herbal remedies with dietary changes that include high-fiber, fermented foods and adequate hydration can significantly improve digestive health. For instance, adding a daily regimen of Fennel tea can complement a diet rich in leafy greens and whole grains, helping to smooth the digestive process and prevent gas build-up. Similarly, incorporating Artichoke leaf extract into a diet low in processed fats can improve fat digestion and prevent the discomfort of a sluggish gallbladder.

So, dear reader, this is your call-to-action to engage in a deeper, more conscious interaction with your body. This approach is not just about alleviating symptoms but about creating a sustainable, harmonious relationship with your digestive system, which has been proven to affect many other aspects of our well-being.

Probiotic Herbs and Prebiotic Foods: Natural Balance for Your Gut

Navigating the intricate world of gut health, you might have encountered the terms 'probiotics' and 'prebiotics,' often used interchangeably yet representing distinctly different components essential for maintaining a healthy gut flora. Probiotics are live microorganisms that, when administered in adequate amounts, confer a health benefit on the host, primarily by enhancing the microbial balance within the gut. These are often referred to as 'good' bacteria and include widely known species like Lactobacillus and Bifidobacterium, which are found in various fermented foods and supplements.

Prebiotics, on the other hand, are a type of non-digestible fiber compound that act as food for these probiotics. They pass through the upper part of the gastrointestinal tract and stimulate the growth or activity of advantageous bacteria that colonize the large bowel by acting as substrate for them. Foods rich in prebiotics include chicory root, garlic, onions, leeks, asparagus, and bananas. The synergy between probiotics and prebiotics can significantly enhance gut health, promoting better digestion, stronger immune function, and even improved mental wellness.

While the term 'probiotic herbs' might seem a bit misleading since herbs themselves do not contain live bacteria, certain herbs are celebrated for their probiotic-like effects in supporting the gut environment conducive to healthy bacterial growth. You will find that dandelion greens are rich in inulin, a type of soluble fiber that acts as a prebiotic, nourishing the gut's beneficial bacteria. Similarly, burdock root offers a wealth of arctiin and lignans, which foster a healthy gut microbiota composition. Adding these herbs to your diet can bolster the effectiveness of the probiotics you consume, ensuring that these beneficial organisms thrive in your gut.

Now, this is important: Incorporating these powerful plants and foods into your daily diet need not be a complex process. Start with something as simple as a morning smoothie that includes a banana, a handful of dandelion greens, and a sprinkle of ground burdock root. This not only kicks off your day with a nutrient-rich meal but also supports your gut health from the first meal. For lunch or dinner, consider a salad dressed with a vinaigrette made from garlic-infused olive oil, another excellent way to integrate prebiotics into your meals. Additionally, incorporating fermented foods like yogurt, kefir, sauerkraut, or kimchi into your meals can introduce beneficial probiotics into your system, enhancing your gut flora balance.

Understanding and applying basic fermentation techniques can also empower you to create probiotic-rich foods at home, which I've found to be a delightful and beneficial endeavor.

Fermentation, a metabolic process that produces chemical changes in organic substrates through the action of enzymes, is largely responsible for the development of probiotics in foods. Starting with something as simple as sauerkraut can be an excellent introduction. This involves shredding cabbage, sprinkling it with salt, and then packing it tightly in a jar until the natural juices submerge the cabbage. The sealed jar is then left at room temperature for several days, allowing the natural fermentation to occur. This yields a delicious product rich in probiotics while giving you a hands-on connection to the food you eat.

Including these practices in your lifestyle will not require drastic changes but rather small, manageable adjustments to your daily habits - you've got this! Gradually introduce more prebiotic-rich foods and fermented products into your diet, which will create a gut environment that supports your overall health and well-being.

Herbal Remedies for Common Digestive Issues

In the dance of daily life, digestive discomforts like indigestion, constipation, and diarrhea can disrupt our rhythm and cloud our days. Fortunately, nature provides plenty of herbal remedies that can alleviate these common troubles, each herb offering its unique method of relief. Through understanding the specific actions and preparing personalized remedies, you will be able to treat and prevent these digestive disturbances, ensuring your digestive system performs its vital functions smoothly and comfortably.

Let's explore some targeted herbal remedies that address these prevalent digestive issues. For indigestion, which often manifests as bloating, pain, or discomfort in the stomach, a soothing tea made from chamomile and fennel can be particularly effective. Chamomile, most commonly known for calming the mind, contains antispasmodic properties that relax the muscles of the digestive tract, easing the contractions that can cause discomfort. Fennel, with its carminative qualities, further aids by reducing gas and bloating. To prepare this tea, steep one teaspoon of chamomile flowers and one teaspoon of crushed fennel seeds in a cup of boiling water for 10 minutes. Straining and drinking this tea slowly after meals can provide immediate relief and aid in the proper digestion of foods.

For those dealing with constipation, an issue often caused by insufficient fiber or fluid intake, or as a side effect of certain medications, senna tea offers a natural laxative effect. However, due to its potent nature, it should be used judiciously. Senna works by stimulating the muscles of the colon, facilitating the easier passage of stool. To prepare senna tea, steep about half a teaspoon of dried senna leaves in hot water for 6-8 minutes. Make a note to start with a small dose to assess your body's reaction, as excessive use can lead to cramping or dependency.

Dealing with diarrhea requires a gentle, nurturing approach, as the body is often in a state of depletion. Blackberry root tea is an excellent remedy due to its astringent properties, which help tighten the tissues of the digestive tract, slowing the movement of excessive fluid. To make this tea, simmer one teaspoon of dried blackberry root in one cup of water for about 10 minutes. This remedy not only helps manage diarrhea but also contains nutrients that aid in recovery post-illness.

Personalizing these remedies according to your individual needs is necessary for their effectiveness and safety. For instance, if you find chamomile too sedative or if you're allergic to it, substituting it with ginger can offer similar digestive benefits without the sedative effect. Similarly, if senna tea proves too strong, incorporating milder laxative herbs like dandelion into your diet can provide gentler relief. It's important to consider personal health conditions and potential interactions with other medications you might be taking. Consulting with a healthcare provider before starting any new herbal regimen is advisable, particularly if you have chronic health issues or are pregnant.

Now, prevention - as they say - is better than cure. Incorporating these herbs into your daily regimen can help maintain digestive health and prevent issues before they start. For example, starting your day with a cup of ginger tea can stimulate digestion and prevent indigestion, while including fiber-rich herbs like psyllium in your diet can help prevent constipation. Regular use of these preventive remedies, combined with a balanced diet and adequate hydration, can keep your digestive system running smoothly, allowing you to enjoy your days without the shadow of digestive discomfort looming over them.

Detoxifying Herbs: Safe Cleansing for Gut Health

Detoxification, a term often surrounded by considerable hype in the wellness community, essentially refers to the body's innate process of neutralizing or eliminating toxins through the liver, kidneys, lungs, lymph, and skin. While the body is naturally equipped to carry out these processes, our modern lifestyle—replete with processed foods, environmental pollutants, and stress—can strain our natural detoxification systems. The concept of using herbs to support detoxification is rooted in enhancing these natural processes without introducing harsh protocols that can often lead to nutrient depletion or imbalance. Keep in mind that detoxification should be approached with an understanding that it is not about purging the body aggressively but supporting it gently to optimize its own ability to cleanse.

In the realm of herbal detoxification, Milk Thistle and Dandelion stand out for their supportive roles. Milk Thistle, with its active compound silymarin, is highly regarded for its hepatoprotective properties. It acts fundamentally by shielding the liver cells from toxins and aiding in the regeneration of damaged liver tissue. It also promotes the liver's natural detoxification processes, helping to clear harmful substances from your body more efficiently. Dandelion, often unjustly pegged as a mere garden weed, offers robust support for both liver and kidney detoxification. Its roots and leaves are rich in antioxidants and compounds that stimulate the production of bile, helping to transport toxins out of the liver.

Moreover, it acts as a diuretic, supporting the kidneys in flushing out waste.

Formulating a gentle detox plan using these herbs involves integrating them into daily routines in a way that supports, rather than shocks, your body. Beginning with Milk Thistle, incorporating a standardized extract of this herb in supplement form can be an effective way to ensure you're receiving its liver-supporting benefits. For Dandelion, both roots and leaves can be used to make a detoxifying herbal tea. Simmering chopped dandelion roots in water for about 10 minutes creates a potent decoction, while steeping the leaves adds a milder but beneficial dimension to your detox tea. Consuming this tea twice a day can gently aid your body's natural detoxification processes without adverse effects.

In addition to these herbal remedies, supporting your detox pathways emphasizes the importance of hydration and light exercise—complementary practices that enhance the detoxifying effects of herbs. Proper hydration is crucial as it aids the kidneys in the filtration of waste from the blood. Aim for at least eight glasses of water daily, more if you are actively detoxing, as this will help facilitate the removal of toxins. Incorporating light exercise such as yoga, walking, or swimming can increase blood circulation and help in the efficient removal of toxins through sweat, respiration, and lymphatic drainage. These activities also boost overall energy levels and help reduce stress, further aiding the detoxification process.

As you consider integrating these practices into your lifestyle, understand that detoxification is not an occasional purge but a daily aspect of healthy living. By supporting your body's natural detox pathways with the right herbs and complementary practices, you're enhancing your ability to detoxify while contributing to a stronger, more resilient system overall. This approach ensures that detoxification becomes a sustainable part of your health regimen, aligned with your body's natural rhythms and needs, to support your daily activities and long-term health goals.

Integrating Herbs into a Gut-Healthy Diet

Within the rich world of nutritional wellness, the role of herbs often resembles that of both a spice and a remedy—enhancing flavors while fortifying our digestive health. A balanced diet, abundant in diverse nutrients, forms the cornerstone of digestive wellness. Yet, the strategic inclusion of specific herbs can elevate this foundation, enhancing the digestive benefits and optimizing gut health. Enriching your meals with digestive-supporting herbs is easy to implement, caters to the palate and also contributes significantly to your gut's functionality and overall health.

When considering the integration of herbs into your daily diet, envision each meal as an opportunity to nourish and heal your body. Herbs like basil, oregano, and thyme, while commonly used for their flavors, also possess remarkable health benefits that target the digestive system. Basil acts as an anti-inflammatory and can help to combat the pain and bloating that often accompany digestive disturbances. Oregano, rich in antioxidants and antibacterial properties, supports gut health by protecting against pathogens. Thyme, with its compounds that relax the intestinal muscles, aids in reducing the discomforts of irritable bowel syndrome (IBS). Incorporating these herbs into your meals is as simple as sprinkling chopped basil over a tomato salad, adding fresh oregano to homemade pizza sauces, or infusing soups and stews with thyme.

Furthermore, the art of meal planning can significantly benefit from the inclusion of these aromatic herbs. Planning meals that incorporate both gut-supportive foods and herbs ensures that every dish contributes positively to your digestive health. One option would be a weekly meal plan that includes a peppermint tea breakfast smoothie to soothe the stomach, a midday salad dressed with lemon and ginger vinaigrette to stimulate digestion, and an evening meal of grilled fish seasoned with fennel for its carminative effects. This approach diversifies your intake of beneficial herbs and helps in maintaining an ongoing enhancement of gut health.

Monitoring the effects of integrating herbs into your diet is essential to understanding their impact on your gut health. Signs of improved digestion might include reduced bloating, a decrease in indigestion episodes, and a more regular bowel movement pattern. Keeping a food diary can be an invaluable tool in this process. By recording what you eat and noting any changes in your digestive health, you can pinpoint which herbs are most beneficial for you and adjust your diet accordingly. This personalized approach will allow you to tailor your herbal intake to your body's unique needs, maximizing the digestive benefits.

EIGHT

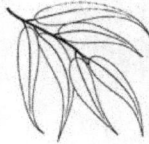

HOLISTIC WELL-BEING

At times, our minds are like a sprawling, twisty garden—some parts blooming with lively ideas, others overrun with the weeds of brain fog (probably planted by too much screen time and not enough sleep). Navigating this mental landscape isn't just a question of determination; it takes clarity, focus, and maybe a little herbal backup.

In a world where information comes at us faster than a runaway herbal tea spill, staying sharp isn't just a perk, it's a necessity. And this is where the magic of plant medicine steps in. Nature has been perfecting its formulas for centuries, and lucky for us, it has gifted us some serious brain-boosting allies. Meet Ginkgo Biloba and Rosemary, your time-tested, science-backed, memory-boosting besties. These herbs have been sharpening minds and kicking brain fog to the curb long before modern distractions took over.

So, grab a cozy cup of tea (preferably with one of these power-houses steeping inside), and let's dive into herbal remedies that will help you think clearer, regulate your emotions, focus better, and maybe even remember where you left your keys.

Herbs for Mental Clarity and Focus

Ginkgo Biloba, often revered as a living fossil, has graced our planet for over 200 million years. Known for its distinctive fan-shaped leaves, this herb has carved its niche not only in time but also in the realm of cognitive enhancement. Traditionally used to ward off the specter of memory loss and support overall brain health, Ginkgo is particularly famed for its ability to improve blood circulation. Enhanced blood flow to the brain means a better supply of oxygen and nutrients, crucial for optimal brain function. Rosemary, on the other hand, is not just for culinary use. This aromatic herb, with its needle-like leaves, has been symbolically and practically linked to remembrance and mental acuity. Its active component, 1,8-cineole, has been shown to increase neurotransmitter activity, thereby boosting memory and alertness.

Mechanisms of Action

THE EFFECTIVENESS of Ginkgo Biloba stems from its rich flavonoid and terpenoid content. These compounds are potent antioxidants that protect neural cells from oxidative stress, a key factor in cognitive decline. Additionally, Ginkgo's ability to modulate neurotransmitter systems enhances neural processing and mental performance. Rosemary's cognitive benefits are primarily attributed to its ability to inhibit acetylcholinesterase, an enzyme that breaks down the neurotransmitter acetylcholine, which is essential for learning and memory. By slowing this breakdown, Rosemary allows for prolonged activity of acetylcholine, enhancing mental clarity and information retention.

Usage Guidelines: Optimal Dosages and Forms

INCORPORATING these herbs into your daily regimen can be both effective and enjoyable. Ginkgo Biloba is most commonly taken in capsule or extract form, with a recommended dosage of 120 to 240 mg per day, ideally starting at the lower end to gauge individual tolerance. For Rosemary, using the fresh or dried herb in cooking is beneficial, but for a more concentrated boost, essential oil or teas are excellent choices. A few drops of Rosemary oil in a diffuser can invigorate the mind during work or study, while a sprig of fresh Rosemary in your tea can provide a mild yet effective cognitive uplift.

Synergizing with Mindfulness and Brain Exercises

To MAXIMIZE the cognitive benefits of these herbs, integrating complementary techniques such as mindfulness and targeted brain exercises can be particularly advantageous. Mindfulness meditation, for instance, enhances focus and reduces stress, creating an optimal mental environment for the herbs to exert their benefits. Simple brain exercises, like crossword puzzles or learning a new language, stimulate neural pathways, increasing mental flexibility and resilience. Combining these practices with regular herbal supplementation creates a holistic approach to cognitive health, ensuring your mind remains as sharp as a tack in a world full of distractions.

Natural Sleep Aids: Herbs for a Restful Night

Navigating the serene world of sleep can often feel like chasing a delicate, elusive butterfly through the hustle and bustle of daily life. In our fast-paced world, the gift of a peaceful night's sleep is something many yearn for yet find just out of reach. This is where the gentle power of herbs like Valerian root and Chamomile can transform our nightly routine, not by force but through a natural easing into the restful embrace of sleep. These herbs, steeped in both tradition and modern research, offer a bridge to the tranquil rest we seek.

Valerian root, with its earthy scent and deep historical roots in herbal medicine, stands out as a beacon for those seeking a sanctuary of sleep. Known for its sedative qualities, Valerian works by subtly increasing the levels of gamma-aminobutyric acid (GABA) in the brain, a neurotransmitter that helps regulate nerve impulses. This action is akin to how certain prescription sleeping pills operate, but Valerian does this gently, without the harsh side effects often associated with pharmaceuticals. Chamomile, a daisy-like herb, offers a milder but equally profound calming effect. Its magic lies in the compound apigenin, which binds to GABA receptors in the brain, promoting relaxation and combating insomnia.

The preparation of these herbs is as important as their selection. For Valerian, a root decoction is effective. This involves simmering the chopped root in water for 10 to 15 minutes, which extracts its active compounds. Straining this mixture into a cup creates a potent brew that's best taken 30 minutes before bedtime. Chamomile, on the other hand, can be enjoyed as a simple tea made by steeping the dried flowers in hot water for about 5 to 7 minutes. This allows for the extraction of essential oils and fills the room with a soothing aroma, enhancing the pre-sleep ritual.

As you can imagine, incorporating these herbs into a comprehensive sleep hygiene practice multiplies their benefits. Sleep hygiene encompasses the various habits and practices that are conducive to sleeping well on a regular basis. This includes maintaining a regular sleep schedule, creating a bedtime ritual that signals to your body that it's time to wind down, and ensuring your sleeping environment is conducive to rest. Integrating Valerian or Chamomile into this routine can enhance these practices, making the transition to sleep smoother and more natural. For instance, sipping Chamomile tea while reading a book in dim light can signal to your body that it is time to slow down, setting the stage for deeper, more restorative sleep.

Personalizing your use of these herbal sleep aids ensures they meet your specific needs and lifestyle. While some may find the strong flavor of Valerian root challenging, combining it with milder flavors like honey or lemon can make the decoction more palatable. Others might prefer the simplicity and mild taste of Chamomile, perhaps adding it to a warm bath before bedtime for a more immersive relaxation experience. Again, listening to your body's responses to these herbs is key; starting with smaller doses and gradually adjusting can help you find the optimum amount that supports your sleep without leaving you feeling groggy in the morning.

In embracing these natural sleep aids, you will reconnect with a traditional wisdom that views sleep as a critical component of health and well-being. As you prepare your nightly cup of Valerian or Chamomile, consider it a most beautiful ritual, a moment to pause and reflect on the day, to release the stresses and to invite calm. This practice prepares your body for sleep, nourishes your soul, reminding you that each night offers a chance to reset, to rest deeply, and to rise refreshed, ready to face the new day with vitality and clarity.

Herbal Support for Energy and Vitality

Within the sometimes-chaotic happenings of our daily responsibilities, maintaining energy levels can often feel like an uphill battle against fatigue and lethargy. It's in these moments that we find ourselves reaching for quick fixes—caffeine, sugar, or other stimulants—that offer a fleeting boost but leave us crashing harder than before. However, nature provides a more sustainable solution through herbs like Ginseng and Rhodiola, which invigorate the body's inherent energy systems without the harsh effects of conventional stimulants. These herbs stand out not only for their efficacy but also for their ability to enhance overall vitality by supporting the body's adrenal health and balancing blood sugar levels.

Ginseng, revered in traditional Chinese medicine for centuries, is often hailed as the king of all tonics. It acts as a natural adaptogen, which means it helps the body adapt to and resist physical, chemical, and biological stressors. By bolstering the adrenal glands, which regulate the stress response and secrete key hormones like adrenaline and cortisol, Ginseng helps sustain energy levels throughout the day. Its impact on blood sugar is equally beneficial; Ginseng promotes the slow and steady release of glucose into the bloodstream, providing a consistent supply of energy without the spikes and crashes associated with sugary snacks.

Rhodiola, another robust adaptogen, thrives in the cold, mountainous regions of Europe and Asia, where its ability to enhance physical and mental endurance has been utilized by mountain communities for generations. Similar to Ginseng, Rhodiola stimulates the body's energy production processes at a cellular level, enhancing mitochondrial function—the powerhouse of the cell—and improving the efficiency of energy utilization. Moreover, Rhodiola has been shown to increase the synthesis of ATP, the primary energy carrier in the body, which plays a crucial role in delivering energy to our cells, tissues, and organs.

Integrating these energy-boosting herbs into your daily routine can be both simple and delightful. Starting your day with a Ginseng-infused morning tonic can invigorate your morning ritual. You can prepare this by steeping Ginseng roots in hot water or adding a few drops of Ginseng tincture to your morning tea. For an afternoon pick-me-up, a Rhodiola tea, made from steeping the dried roots in hot water, can be a perfect replacement for your usual cup of coffee. These small, consistent incorporations not only boost energy levels but also integrate the adaptogenic benefits of these herbs into your life, helping you manage stress and maintain vitality.

The synergy between these energizing herbs and lifestyle choices cannot be overstated. Regular physical activity, for instance, naturally increases energy levels and is complemented by the stamina-enhancing properties of Ginseng and Rhodiola. Incorporating moderate exercise into your routine, such as a daily walk or a morning yoga session, can amplify the effects of these herbs, creating a cycle of enhanced energy and health. Stress management, another crucial aspect of maintaining energy levels, is also supported by adaptogens. Techniques like mindfulness meditation or deep breathing exercises can reduce stress-induced fatigue, and when paired with adaptogenic herbs, they provide a robust defense against the draining effects of stress.

Aging Gracefully with Herbs: Natural Antioxidants and Anti-Inflammatories

As the years advance, the quest for vitality and youthfulness remains a constant, prompting many to explore avenues that promise to ease the signs of aging. In this exploration, nature offers its bounty in the form of herbs like Turmeric and Green Tea, renowned for their culinary merits and their profound anti-aging benefits. These herbs are steeped in antioxidant and anti-inflammatory properties, which play a central role in mitigating the cellular wear and tear that accompanies aging. Turmeric, with its vibrant golden hue, contains curcumin, a compound that has been extensively studied for its antioxidant abilities. It helps in neutralizing free radicals—molecules that cause oxidative stress and damage to cells, accelerating the aging process. Green Tea, rich in catechins like EGCG (epigallocatechin gallate), offers similar benefits, reducing inflammation and protecting cells from damage that can lead to premature aging and various diseases.

The skin, our largest organ, often reflects our overall health and is the most visible indicator of age. Both Turmeric and Green Tea contribute significantly to skin health by enhancing elasticity and brightness while reducing inflammation that can cause skin issues such as eczema and rosacea. These herbs support the skin's ability to repair itself from the inside out, promoting a healthy glow that transcends cosmetic enhancements. For instance, the topical application of Turmeric in the form of a face mask can reduce the appearance of wrinkles and fine lines by improving collagen synthesis, which is vital for maintaining the skin's structural integrity. Similarly, rinsing your face with Green Tea or applying it as a toner can diminish puffiness and redness, thanks to its anti-inflammatory properties.

Preparing these herbs for use in your skincare routine can be both a therapeutic and creative endeavor. A simple Turmeric face mask can be made by mixing turmeric powder with honey, a natural humectant, and a bit of Greek yogurt for its soothing properties. Apply this mixture to your face for about 15 minutes before rinsing with warm water to reveal refreshed and revitalized skin. For Green Tea, brewing a strong cup and allowing it to cool can serve as an excellent base for a homemade toner. Mixing this tea with aloe vera gel and a few drops of vitamin E oil creates a soothing, antioxidative toner that can be applied with a cotton ball after cleansing.

Taking a holistic approach to aging involves more than just addressing skin health; it encompasses fostering well-being across mental, physical, and emotional domains. Integrating Turmeric and Green Tea into your daily diet can amplify their health benefits. For example, starting your day with a warm cup of Green Tea can boost your antioxidant intake, providing cellular protection throughout the day. Adding Turmeric to your meals, whether in curries, soups, or as a spice in vegetable sautés, can similarly enhance your diet with anti-inflammatory benefits. This daily integration helps in managing many physical symptoms of aging while supporting cognitive functions and emotional health, contributing to a balanced and vibrant life as the years advance.

In addition to dietary integration, combining the use of these herbs with lifestyle practices that promote overall health can profoundly impact how gracefully one ages. Regular physical activity, adequate hydration, and stress management are all enhanced by the regular intake of these antioxidative and anti-inflammatory herbs. Yoga and meditation, for example, not only reduce stress but also improve physical flexibility and mental clarity, qualities that are essential for maintaining vitality at any age. When paired with a diet rich in herbs like Turmeric and Green Tea, these practices form a comprehensive approach to aging that supports longevity and enhances the quality of life, allowing you to embrace each year with health, happiness, and grace.

Herbs for Hormonal Balance

Navigating the shifts in life's seasons, especially during menopause, can often feel like steering through uncharted waters. As you face the complexities of hormonal changes, the discomforts of hot flashes, night sweats, and mood swings may seem daunting. Yet, with herbal medicine, we find gentle, natural allies like Black Cohosh and Red Clover, which can offer some much-needed relief during these turbulent times. These herbs, deeply rooted in traditional practices and supported by modern research, provide hope and balance, helping to smooth the transition through menopause and beyond.

Black Cohosh, an herb native to North America, has been a cornerstone in indigenous medicine and is widely used today for its effectiveness in easing menopausal symptoms. Its ability to mimic estrogen is particularly beneficial, as it fills the hormonal gaps naturally occurring during menopause, thus alleviating hot flashes and improving mood stability. This herb acts primarily through its influence on serotonin receptors, which play a crucial role in regulating body temperature and mood. The modulation of these receptors can help stabilize the body's response to the declining estrogen levels seen in menopause, providing a sense of equilibrium during this phase of life.

Red Clover, another phytoestrogen-rich herb, complements Black Cohosh by providing additional support for hormonal balance. Rich in isoflavones, a type of phytoestrogen, Red Clover helps manage the intensity and frequency of hot flashes and also supports cardiovascular health, which can be a concern as estrogen levels decline. Its gentle action on the hormonal system makes it a valuable herb for long-term use, contributing to symptom relief as well as overall vitality and wellness post-menopause.

Now, the safe usage of these herbs is paramount, especially

considering their interactions with hormone replacement therapies (HRT). While Black Cohosh and Red Clover can offer significant benefits, it's crucial to consult with a healthcare provider to understand their suitability for your specific health profile, particularly if you are undergoing HRT. These herbs should complement, not replace, prescribed treatments unless advised by a professional. Starting with lower doses and gradually adjusting based on your body's responses allows for a personalized approach to herbal supplementation, minimizing any risks and maximizing the benefits.

Expanding the scope beyond menopause, the benefits of hormonal balance achieved through these herbs extend into broader aspects of health. Maintaining hormonal equilibrium can influence various body systems, potentially reducing the risk of chronic conditions associated with post-menopausal years, such as osteoporosis and heart disease. The anti-inflammatory properties of Red Clover and the adaptogenic effects of Black Cohosh can play roles in this broader health context, supporting hormonal health and enhancing overall resilience.

Of course, incorporating these herbs into your daily regimen will require thoughtful consideration of both form and timing. Teas, tinctures, and capsules offer various ways of consuming Black Cohosh and Red Clover, with tinctures and capsules generally providing a more concentrated and controlled dosage. Integrating these into your morning or evening routine can help establish consistent use, which is key to achieving their full therapeutic potential. Additionally, lifestyle factors such as a balanced diet rich in calcium and regular physical activity should act in concert with these herbal therapies to support bone density and heart health, further enriching your post-menopausal years.

Herbal First Aid: Quick Remedies for Minor Injuries and Ailments

In the comforting embrace of your home or while adventuring in the great outdoors, minor injuries and ailments can suddenly arise, turning tranquil moments into sources of stress and discomfort. Fortunately, nature provides an abundance of herbal allies, such as Calendula and Aloe Vera, ready to soothe cuts, bruises, burns, and more. These plants have stood the test of time, not only for their effectiveness but also for their safety, making them ideal components of a natural first aid kit. This approach to first aid will empower you to handle common minor injuries with confidence while aligning with a holistic perspective on health, where nature's bounty is a first resort in nurturing well-being.

Calendula, with its brilliant orange blossoms, is celebrated for its anti-inflammatory and antimicrobial properties, making it an excellent herb for treating cuts and bruises. The flavonoids and carotenoids present in Calendula contribute to its ability to speed up wound healing and reduce inflammation, providing relief and reducing the risk of infection. Aloe Vera, known for its thick, succulent leaves, contains a gel that is a soothing balm for burns. Rich in glycoproteins and polysaccharides, Aloe Vera gel helps to reduce pain and inflammation while promoting skin repair and hydration. Preparing these remedies is straightforward and can be done with minimal tools and ingredients, ensuring they are accessible whenever needed.

To harness the benefits of Calendula, creating a simple salve can be an effective way to apply its healing properties directly to the skin. This can be done by infusing Calendula petals in a carrier oil, such as coconut or olive oil, over low heat for several hours. After straining out the petals, the infused oil can be mixed with beeswax to form a salve, which can be stored in small jars or tins. This salve can be applied to cuts or bruises, forming a protective layer that aids in healing and prevents infection. Aloe Vera gel can be used directly from the plant by slicing a leaf open and applying the fresh gel to a burn, offering immediate cooling relief and speeding up the skin's healing process.

Assembling an herbal first aid kit is a proactive step towards being prepared for common injuries. Essential items for this kit include

Calendula salve, Aloe Vera gel, and other herbal remedies such as lavender essential oil for its calming and antiseptic properties, and tea tree oil, known for its broad-spectrum antimicrobial activity. These can be complemented with practical tools like bandages, cotton swabs, and tweezers, so that you have a well-rounded kit ready at a moment's notice. Keep it in an easily accessible location at home. You might also want a portable version in your car or backpack when traveling, to ensure that you are always prepared to handle minor injuries effectively and naturally.

It's crucial, however, to recognize the limitations of herbal first aid. While effective for minor injuries and ailments, more severe conditions such as deep cuts, persistent burns, or infections require professional medical attention. Herbal remedies can provide initial care but are not substitutes for comprehensive medical treatment when it's needed.

Don't forget that understanding when to seek professional help is just as important as knowing how to use herbal remedies; it is our own responsibility to make sure that we are using these natural tools responsibly and effectively.

Let me tell you: There is something highly empowering about embracing a form of preparedness that is grounded in natural care and self-reliance. Although this is merely an overview of natural alternatives, I hope it equips you with the knowledge to handle minor injuries and, once more, deepen your connection to the healing powers of nature. These practices are sure to increase your confidence and competence in natural health practices.

NINE

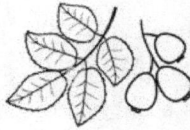

HERBAL HACKS BEYOND THE BASICS

So, you've mastered the herbal basics: infusions, tinctures, maybe even a salve or two. You know your chamomile from your calendula and can whip up an immune-boosting tea like a kitchen witch on a mission. But now, it's time to level up. In this chapter, we will be diving into the next stage of herbal mastery—the kind of techniques that take your remedies from "Hey, this works!" to "Whoa, is this *magic*?" (Spoiler: It's just really good science, but we can pretend.)

We're talking about refined extraction methods, potency-boosting techniques, and the little-known tricks that make your herbal creations even more effective. It's a path that requires a bit more patience and precision, but trust me, the rewards are worth it.

Mastering Herbal Extracts: Advanced Techniques for Potency

The journey of an herbalist is ever-evolving, and mastering advanced extraction methods such as percolation and Soxhlet extraction marks a significant milestone. Percolation, though less commonly practiced by casual herbal enthusiasts, is a dynamic method for extracting herbal constituents quickly and efficiently. Imagine it as brewing coffee, where the solvent passes through a column of finely ground herbs, pulling out the active compounds with remarkable efficacy. The result? A potent, concentrated extract in a fraction of the time it takes for maceration.

Soxhlet extraction takes it a step further. This method, typically used in scientific labs, involves continuously boiling and condensing a solvent, which then washes over the plant material, extracting compounds with each cycle. While more complex, the beauty of Soxhlet extraction lies in its ability to thoroughly extract constituents until the solvent can dissolve no more, ensuring that no active component is left behind. These techniques, while advanced, open up a new dimension of potency and precision in herbal preparation that can significantly enhance the therapeutic value of your remedies.

Solvent Selection

IN THE ART OF EXTRACTION, choosing the right solvent is as important as the process itself. The solvent acts as a carrier that absorbs and holds onto the desired herbal constituents. Common solvents include alcohol, glycerine, water, and vinegar, each serving a specific purpose and extracting different types of substances. Alcohol, for example, is excellent for extracting a wide range of compounds, including alkaloids, flavonoids, and volatile oils. It is also a preservative, which extends the shelf life of your extracts. Glycerine offers a sweeter taste and is preferable for creating alcohol-free products, ideal for children and those avoiding alcohol for health or personal reasons. Water, the solvent for teas and decoctions, is universally available but extracts a more limited range of compounds. Vinegar, rich in acetic acid, is excellent for minerals and other alkaline elements.

When selecting a solvent, consider not just the solubility of the active compounds but also the intended use of the extract. The choice of solvent affects everything from the extract's potency to its shelf life and suitability for various age groups or health conditions. Understanding the properties and limitations of each solvent will allow you to tailor your extracts to meet specific needs, enhancing both their effectiveness and applicability.

Standardization vs. Whole Herb Extracts

THE DEBATE between using standardized extracts and whole herb extracts is at the heart of modern herbal practice. Standardized extracts aim for consistency, with a specific, quantified amount of certain active compounds in each batch. This method appeals to those who seek predictability in their herbal remedies, ensuring that each dose delivers a precise amount of active ingredients. However, whole herb extracts celebrate the natural complexity of plants. They contain the full spectrum of a plant's constituents, working synergistically—the way nature intended—to provide a balanced, holistic effect. This approach is often favored in traditional herbal medicine, where the interplay of multiple compounds is considered essential for the remedy's full therapeutic effect.

Preservation and Storage

PRESERVING the potency of herbal extracts is as crucial as their preparation. Proper storage conditions can significantly extend the life and effectiveness of your extracts. Dark glass containers are ideal for protecting sensitive compounds from light degradation. Keeping these containers in a cool, dry place helps prevent the degradation of active ingredients. For extracts not inherently preserved by their solvent, such as those in water, refrigeration may be necessary to prevent spoilage. Additionally, incorporating oxygen absorbers into storage containers can further protect against oxidative degradation, ensuring that your extracts remain as potent as the day they were made.

All of these methods combined - both simple and complex - are so much more than just procedures; they are unique transformations, ways to unlock the deeper potential of plants, bringing forth their fullest therapeutic powers.

Your journey with herbs is one of continuous learning and discovery, and mastering these advanced techniques will expand your horizons within the art and science of herbal medicine.

Phytochemistry: Understanding Plant Compounds

Each and every phytochemical is unique and essential for the life-sustaining properties of plants. As we look into this fascinating subject, you'll discover that these natural compounds are not just biochemical constituents but rather comprise the very essence of a plant's interaction with our body, contributing to health and protection against diseases. Phytochemistry is the study of these compounds extracted from plants, and understanding their roles and actions can significantly enhance your ability to use herbs effectively.

Phytochemicals, ranging from well-known flavonoids and terpenes to lesser-known but equally vital saponins and glycosides, play diverse roles. They can act as antioxidants, protecting cells from oxidative stress; as anti-inflammatory agents, reducing swelling and pain; or as adaptogens, helping the body manage stress. Others might exhibit antibacterial or antiviral properties, making them valuable in fighting infections. Each phytochemical interacts with the human body in complex ways, often binding to or modulating the function of specific enzymes and receptors, influencing well-being at a cellular level.

The process of analyzing these phytochemicals involves sophisticated techniques that ensure the identification and quantification of these compounds in various herbs. Chromatography, a method used extensively in phytochemical analysis, involves the separation of a mixture into its components based on differences in their affinity to a stationary phase and a mobile phase. Techniques such as gas chromatography (GC) and high-performance liquid chromatography (HPLC) are particularly useful for isolating volatile and non-volatile compounds, respectively. Spectrophotometry, another critical analytical technique, measures how much light a substance absorbs. It is instrumental in determining the concentration of phytochemicals, particularly those with antioxidant properties, by measuring light absorption at specific wavelengths.

Understanding the interactions among various phytochemicals within a single plant or herbal blend can make a difference in our approach to herbal medicine. The concept of entourage effect – a fascinating topic - proposes that these compounds do not act in isolation but synergistically enhance each other's effects. For instance, the anti-inflammatory action of one phytochemical may be enhanced by the antioxidant activity of another, providing a combined effect greater than the sum of their individual actions. This holistic interaction can lead to more effective remedies, highlighting the importance of using whole herb extracts in some therapeutic contexts as opposed to isolated active ingredients.

Yet, with great potency comes great responsibility. Safety considerations are paramount when dealing with powerful phytochemicals. While many plant compounds offer health benefits, others can be toxic or cause adverse effects if used improperly. Knowledge of an herb's phytochemical profile can guide its safe use, indicating which parts of the plant are safe to use and in what quantities. For instance, certain compounds might be hepatotoxic in large doses or could interact adversely with pharmaceutical medications. Understanding these properties ensures that the use of herbal remedies remains most effective and safe.

Observing the complexities of phytochemistry certainly requires a keen understanding of chemistry. However, even as beginners, we can explore aspects of this topic by falling back on our deep respect for the natural potency of plants. As you continue to explore the relationships between plants and their chemical compounds, you'll likely find yourself even more in awe of the natural world and its sophisticated mechanisms for health and healing.

Creating Personalized Herbal Formulas

When you step into the realm of creating personalized herbal formulas, you embrace a process that is both an art and a science. It begins with a thorough assessment of individual health needs, which is as crucial as the formulation itself. Imagine sitting down with a map before a journey, plotting out your route based on your starting point and destination. Similarly, in herbal formulation, understanding a person's current health status, medical history, lifestyle, and wellness goals allows you to tailor an herbal remedy that precisely meets their needs. This assessment is just as much about noting symptoms as it is about understanding the whole person, which includes diet, stress levels, and even emotional health.

Once you have a clear picture of the individual's health landscape, the next step is the formulation of the herbal blend. This is where your knowledge of herbology comes into play. As you now know, each herb offers a unique combination of benefits and knowing how to combine them can amplify their effects. For instance, if you're creating a blend to help with sleep, you might start with a base of chamomile for its calming properties, then add valerian root for its stronger sedative effects, and perhaps a touch of lavender to enhance the blend's soothing aroma. The key here is balance—ensuring that each herb contributes to the desired outcome without overwhelming the others.

Balancing Tastes and Energetics

IN TRADITIONAL HERBAL MEDICINE, the balance of tastes and energetics within a formula is essential for its effectiveness. The tastes—sweet, sour, bitter, pungent, astringent, and salty—each have their own therapeutic properties. For example, bitter herbs like dandelion can stimulate digestion, while pungent herbs such as ginger can warm the body and break down accumulation. The energetics—hot, cold, dry, moist—also play a crucial role. A person with a cold, sluggish system may benefit from warming herbs like cinnamon, whereas someone with signs of heat and inflammation might need cooling herbs like peppermint.

This nuanced approach ensures that the formula addresses the specific symptoms while harmonizing with the person's overall constitution, promoting deeper, more lasting healing. It's similar to cooking a complex dish, where the flavors need to be balanced so no single taste overwhelms the others, creating a harmonious and satisfying final product.

Dosage and Delivery Methods

DETERMINING the appropriate dosage and delivery method is critical to the success of an herbal formula. Dosages will vary depending on the strength of the herbs, the conditions being treated, and the individual's sensitivity and response to the herbs. For instance, tinctures are often more concentrated and are absorbed more quickly by the body than teas, which might be preferred for their gentler effect and ritualistic aspect of preparation and consumption.

The choice between teas, tinctures, capsules, and powders largely depends on the person's lifestyle and preferences. A busy professional might prefer the convenience of capsules or tinctures, which don't require preparation time and can be easily carried and consumed throughout the day. In contrast, someone who values the ritual of preparing and enjoying a warm cup of herbal tea might favor this traditional method, which can enhance the therapeutic experience through its soothing preparation process.

. . .

Monitoring and Adjusting

THE FINAL STEP in personalized herbal formulation is monitoring and adjusting. This dynamic process is crucial because it considers that the individual's needs may change over time. Regular check-ins to discuss the effects of the herbal formula, any side effects, or changes in health status are imperative. This feedback allows for adjustments to the dosage, formulation, or method of delivery, ensuring the herbal treatment remains aligned with the individual's evolving health needs.

This ongoing monitoring and adjusting process reflects the personalized nature of herbal medicine, where treatments are not static but adaptive, tailored continuously to fit the individual as they move through different stages of health and life. It's a process that requires patience, observation, and responsiveness—qualities that define the most skilled herbal practitioners. Developing your ability to create and refine herbal formulas will allow you to develop your expertise whilst deepening your connection to the healing power of nature.

Navigating Herb-Drug Interactions

Within the intricacies of integrating herbal remedies with conventional medications, understanding the nuances of herb-drug interactions is crucial. These interactions occur because many herbs and pharmaceuticals share metabolic pathways in the body, primarily involving liver enzymes responsible for drug metabolism. Enzymes such as Cytochrome P450 play a pivotal role here; they metabolize drugs, and their activity can be inhibited or induced by certain herbal constituents. For example, St. John's Wort is known to induce these enzymes, potentially reducing the effectiveness of medications such as antidepressants and birth control pills by increasing their metabolic rate. Conversely, herbs like Grapefruit can inhibit these enzymes, leading to decreased metabolism of drugs like statins, increasing their blood levels and potential toxicity.

The implications of such interactions are significant, ranging from diminished drug efficacy to unexpected side effects, which can compromise your health care. Therefore, being well-informed about these interactions is not just beneficial—it's a necessity for anyone integrating herbal therapies with conventional treatments. Highlighting common interactions helps in anticipating and managing potential risks. For instance, Warfarin, a commonly prescribed anticoagulant, can have its effects potentiated by herbs like Ginkgo biloba, leading to an increased risk of bleeding. Similarly, the sedative effects of pharmaceuticals like benzodiazepines can be enhanced by herbal sedatives such as Valerian root, potentially leading to excessive sedation.

Managing these risks involves a proactive, informed approach. Keeping abreast of the latest research is vital, as new interactions can be identified as more is understood about both herbal and pharmaceutical metabolisms. Implementing a thorough patient history taking is equally crucial. This should include a detailed account of all the medications, both herbal and pharmaceutical, that you are taking. Understanding your complete medication profile allows for a critical evaluation of potential interactions and their management strategies. These strategies might include adjusting medication timings, modifying doses, or, in some cases, substituting or discontinuing an herb or drug to avoid adverse interactions.

Perhaps the most crucial aspect in managing herb-drug interactions is fostering open communication lines between you, your herbalist, and your healthcare provider. This triad forms the cornerstone of safe and effective healthcare management. You are encouraged to discuss any herbal supplements you are taking, just as you would discuss your conventional medications. This transparency allows healthcare providers to give you the best possible care, considering all aspects of your health regimen. It also provides an opportunity for healthcare providers to educate themselves and their patients about the benefits and risks associated with herbal medicines. Open dialogue not only helps in managing health effectively but also in building trust and confidence in the therapeutic process. It ensures that all parties are informed and in agreement with the treatment plan, which enhances adherence to prescribed therapies and leads to better health outcomes.

The Future of Herbal Medicine: Trends and Innovations

As we explore the horizon of herbal medicine, it becomes increasingly clear that this field is poised at the cusp of significant transformation, driven by advances in research and technology. The exploration of new medicinal plants and the application of genomic studies are expanding our understanding of plant-based therapies, revealing the potential for new herbal remedies and offering deeper insights into the ancient wisdom that has guided herbal practices for centuries. These cutting-edge research initiatives are key as they help in identifying genetic markers that influence plant behavior under various environmental stresses, thereby aiding in the cultivation of more potent medicinal plants.

Moreover, the integration of high-throughput screening methods is revolutionizing the way active compounds are identified in herbs. This technology allows for rapid testing of thousands of samples simultaneously, significantly speeding up the discovery process and helping researchers pinpoint which components of a plant are responsible for its therapeutic effects. Furthermore, the advent of artificial intelligence (AI) in herbal medicine is transforming formulation strategies. AI algorithms can analyze vast amounts of data on herbal efficacy and safety, predicting how different herbal combinations might interact. This enhances the precision of herbal remedies while personalizing them to an individual's unique health profile, marking a shift towards more tailored and effective treatments.

Sustainability and ethical sourcing in the herbal medicine

sector are receiving increased attention as the global demand for herbal products continues to grow. The sustainability of plant resources is vital, ensuring that their use today does not compromise their availability for future generations. Ethical sourcing, on the other hand, involves procuring herbs in a way that is fair to both the environment and the communities involved in their cultivation and harvest. This includes fair trade practices that ensure farmers and gatherers are compensated fairly and working conditions that respect human rights. The importance of these practices cannot be overstated, as they directly impact the quality of herbal products and the lives of those who depend on this industry for their livelihood.

The potential for greater integration of herbal medicine into mainstream healthcare systems also presents a promising frontier. This integration faces several challenges, including regulatory obstacles and the need for more professional training opportunities in herbal medicine within conventional medical education. However, the benefits of such integration could be profound, offering patients more diverse treatment options that combine the best of both conventional and herbal medicine. Efforts to standardize herbal medicine practices and ensure their safety and efficacy through rigorous clinical trials and quality controls are important steps toward this integration. These efforts help in building trust among healthcare providers and patients and facilitate a more holistic approach to health care, where the natural and conventional modalities complement each other efficiently.

As you consider these advancements and look towards the future, remember that the field of herbal medicine is not just evolving; it is thriving. It continues to grow richer with every research breakthrough and technological innovation, promising a future where herbal remedies are not seen merely as alternatives but as integral components of a comprehensive approach to health and wellness. The journey through the landscape of herbal medicine is one of endless discovery. It offers a beautiful blend of tradition and innovation, where each new finding enhances our connection to the natural world and our understanding of its capacity to heal.

Building Your Herbal Community

When it comes to health and holistic well-being, the strength of community cannot be overstated. Connecting with fellow herbalists, healers, and enthusiasts can deeply enrich our own practice, as well as strengthen the collective knowledge and advocacy of the herbal community. Engaging with others can be incredibly rewarding, offering opportunities for learning, sharing, and growth.

The first step in building your herbal community is to actively seek networking opportunities. Joining herbal associations is a fantastic way to start. Organizations like the American Herbalists Guild provide a platform for meeting peers who share your passion for plant-based healing. These associations often host conferences, workshops, and seminars that not only serve as learning hubs but also as social gatherings where you can meet and mingle with like-minded individuals. Additionally, in today's digital age, online forums and social media groups play a central role. Platforms such as Herb-Mentor offer courses, resources, and forums where beginners and seasoned practitioners exchange ideas, advice, and encouragement.

Once you've made connections, engaging in collaborative projects can be a fulfilling way to contribute to the herbal community. Participating in or initiating community gardens that focus on medicinal plants creates a space for communal learning and sharing of herbal knowledge. Similarly, joining or establishing herbal medicine co-ops where remedies and resources can be shared or traded can help build a supportive network. These projects help foster community spirit while promoting sustainable practices within herbal medicine, as they encourage the local cultivation and use of medicinal plants.

Mentorship and Education

EDUCATION IS A LIFELONG PROCESS, especially in a field as ever-evolving as herbal medicine. Seeking mentorship from experienced practitioners can dramatically enhance your learning curve. Whether through formal apprenticeships or informal mentorship arrangements, learning from seasoned herbalists can provide you with insights and knowledge that are not found in books or online courses. On the flip side, if you are an experienced practitioner, offering mentorship to novices can be immensely rewarding and vital for the continued growth and vitality of the herbal community. Additionally, pursuing advanced courses in herbal medicine not only broadens your own knowledge but also prepares you to contribute more effectively to community education and projects.

Advocacy and Activism

AS HERBALISTS, you have the unique opportunity to advocate for the wider acceptance and integration of herbal medicine into mainstream healthcare. This involves not only promoting the efficacy and safety of herbal treatments but also advocating for the preservation of traditional plant knowledge and sustainable practices within the industry. Participation in policy reform discussions, community health initiatives, and public seminars can elevate the role of herbal medicine in public health. By raising awareness and disseminating accurate information, you help pave the way for a healthcare paradigm that acknowledges and incorporates the holistic benefits of herbal medicine.

Reflection

ENGAGING with the herbal community is not just about enhancing your own practice; it involves contributing to a collective movement that values sustainable, holistic health solutions. Each connection you make, each project you participate in, and each initiative you support adds to the strength and richness of this community, driving forward the integration of herbal medicine into broader health practices and enriching lives with the healing power of plants.

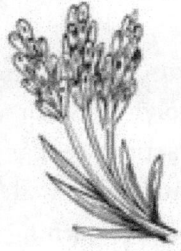

Take a moment to reflect on your current role within the herbal community. Are you more of a learner, seeking knowledge and mentorship, or are you ready to share your expertise and mentor others? How can you engage more actively in advocacy or collaborative projects?

Jot down your thoughts and goals to help clarify your path forward and identify areas where you can make a meaningful impact.

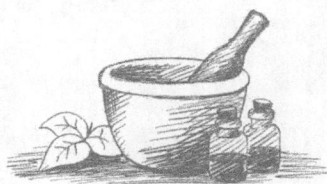

ESSENTIAL NATURAL REMEDIES

66 Nature itself is the best physician.

HIPPOCRATES

Take a breath. Close your eyes. Imagine, for a moment, stepping into a serene sanctuary where every shelf and cupboard holds the secrets to natural health and wellness.

Here, in this special chapter, we'll step into this unique apothecary store. I have decided to unveil my fifteen favorite natural concoctions – all of which are simple, natural, and profoundly effective. Each one possesses a natural healing power; get ready to soothe, heal, and rejuvenate both mind and body. These are remedies passed down through generations, backed by both traditional wisdom and modern research, ready to be rediscovered and integrated into your daily routine.

HERBAL HACKS FOR BODY & MIND

Ginger and Honey Tea

A staple in many households for its soothing properties, this tea is a powerhouse for easing digestion and boosting the immune system. Ginger is known for its warming and anti-inflammatory properties, for stimulating digestive enzymes, enhancing the absorption of nutrients and relieving gastrointestinal distress. Honey, rich in antioxidants, lends not only sweetness but also an antibacterial boost, making this tea a comforting ally during cold and flu season.

Ingredients: 1 cup water, 1-2 inches fresh ginger root, 1 tablespoon honey.

Optional: lemon slices

Procedure:

1. Peel and thinly slice the ginger root.

2. Bring the water to a boil in a small pot.

3. Add the ginger slices to the boiling water.

4. Reduce the heat and let it simmer for about 10 minutes.

5. Remove from heat and strain the tea into a cup.

6. Stir in the honey and add lemon slices if desired.

Enjoy the tea while it's warm.

Lavender Infused Oil

Transitioning from the spicy kick of ginger to the calming embrace of lavender, this versatile elixir is most excellent for stress relief. Used in massages, it can significantly reduce physical and emotional stress, promoting a sense of peace and relaxation. If you are prone to headaches and migraines, this infusion will certainly come in handy. Lavender's ability to lower cortisol levels makes it a go-to remedy for those seeking a natural way to unwind and destress. This oil can also be dabbed on temples or wrists during hectic days or before sleep, providing a gentle, soothing touch that eases the mind into a state of calm.

Ingredients: 1 cup carrier oil (e.g., olive oil, coconut oil, or almond oil), 1/2 cup dried lavender flowers.

Procedure:
1. Place the dried lavender flowers in a clean, dry glass jar.

2. Pour the carrier oil over the lavender flowers, making sure they are fully submerged.

3. Seal the jar tightly and place it in a sunny windowsill.

4. Let the mixture infuse for about 4-6 weeks, shaking the jar occasionally.

5. After the infusion period, strain the oil through a cheesecloth or fine-mesh strainer into a clean bottle.

6. Store the lavender-infused oil in a cool, dark place.

Chamomile and Mint Tea

For those nights when sleep seems just out of reach, a cup of this herbal tea might be the gentle nudge your body needs. Chamomile, known for its mild sedative effects, pairs beautifully with mint, which aids digestion and adds a refreshing flavor. This combination will sooth the stomach and calm the mind, making it easier to slip into a peaceful sleep. It's a simple ritual that can transform your evening routine, providing a much-needed moment of tranquility in your busy life.

Ingredients: 1 tsp dried chamomile flowers, 1 tsp dried mint leaves, 1 cup boiling water.

Procedure: Bring the water to a boil. Place the chamomile flowers and mint leaves in a teapot or cup. Pour the boiling water over the chamomile and mint. Cover and let it steep for about 5-7 minutes. Strain the tea into a cup. Add honey or lemon if desired.

Peppermint and Eucalyptus Inhaler

In moments when the air feels heavy and your mind foggy, reach for this homemade inhaler. The dynamic duo clears the nasal passages and invigorates the senses. Peppermint offers a cooling sensation that can alleviate headaches and respiratory congestion, while eucalyptus has components that fight respiratory infections and ease breathing. Together, they create a refreshing experience that can lift your spirits and sharpen your focus, making it an excellent tool for midday rejuvenation.

Ingredients: 5-10 drops peppermint essential oil, 5-10 drops eucalyptus essential oil, 1 inhaler tube (available at health stores or online). Cotton wick (comes with the inhaler tube).

Procedure:
  1. Place the cotton wick in a small bowl or dish.

2. Add the peppermint and eucalyptus essential oils to the cotton wick, allowing it to soak in.

3. Carefully insert the cotton wick into the inhaler tube.

4. Close the inhaler tube tightly.

5. Use the inhaler by holding it up to your nose and inhaling deeply.

Lemon and Ginger Drink

Served warmed or chilled, this zesty remedy is made to fortify your immune defenses while providing a tangy treat. Lemon, packed with vitamin C, enhances your immune system's ability to fight off infections, while ginger adds a spicy layer of protection with its antiviral properties. This drink wards off colds while stimulating circulation, ensuring that your energy levels are maintained throughout the day. It's a bold concoction that embodies the essence of preventive health care—delicious, simple, and incredibly effective.

Ingredients: 1 cup water, 1-2 inches fresh ginger root, juice of 1 lemon, 1 tablespoon honey, lemon slices or mint leaves for garnish (optional).

Procedure:

1. Peel and thinly slice the ginger root.

2. Bring the water to a boil in a small pot.

3. Add the ginger slices to the boiling water.

4. Reduce the heat and let it simmer for about 10 minutes.

5. Remove from heat and strain the drink into a cup.

6. Stir in the lemon juice and honey.

7. Add lemon slices or mint leaves for garnish if desired.

Enjoy the drink while it's warm or let it cool and enjoy it cold.

Ashwagandha Milk

This blend helps to reduce stress and anxiety, improve sleep, and boost overall vitality. It also supports immune function and enhances memory and cognitive function.

Ingredients: 1 cup milk (dairy or plant-based), 1 teaspoon ashwagandha powder, 1/2 teaspoon turmeric powder (optional), 1/2 teaspoon cinnamon powder (optional), 1-2 teaspoons honey or maple syrup (optional, for sweetness), a pinch of black pepper (optional, to enhance absorption of turmeric), a small piece of fresh ginger or 1/4 teaspoon ginger powder (optional).

Procedure:

1. Heat the Milk: Pour the milk into a small saucepan and heat over medium heat until it begins to simmer. Do not let it boil.

2. Add Ashwagandha Powder: Stir in the ashwagandha powder, ensuring it is well mixed with the milk.

3. Optional Ingredients: If using turmeric, cinnamon, black pepper, and ginger, add them to the milk and stir well.

4. Simmer: Allow the mixture to simmer on low heat for 5-10 minutes. This helps to infuse the milk with the herbs and spices.

5. Sweeten: If desired, add honey or maple syrup to taste and stir until dissolved.

6. Strain (if needed): If you've used fresh ginger or any coarse spices, you may want to strain the milk before serving.

7. Serve: Pour the ashwagandha milk into a cup and enjoy it warm!

Golden Milk

Golden milk has powerful anti-inflammatory and antioxidant properties, supports joint health, improves digestion, and boosts the immune system.

Ingredients: 1 tsp turmeric powder, 1/4 teaspoon ground cinnamon, 1 cup warm milk (dairy or plant-based, such as almond, coconut, or soy milk), pinch of black pepper (to enhance the absorption of turmeric), honey or maple syrup to taste.

Procedure:

1. Heat the Milk: Pour the milk into a small saucepan and heat over medium heat until it begins to simmer. Do not let it boil.

2. Add Spices: Stir in the turmeric, ginger, cinnamon, and black pepper. If using fresh ginger, grate it finely before adding.

3. Simmer: Allow the mixture to simmer on low heat for about 5-10 minutes. This helps to infuse the milk with the spices. Stir occasionally to ensure the spices are well mixed.

4. Sweeten: If desired, add honey or maple syrup to taste and stir until dissolved.

5. Optional Ingredients: For additional flavor, add vanilla extract, cardamom, or nutmeg and stir well.

6. Strain (if needed): If you've used fresh ginger or any coarse spices, you may want to strain the milk before serving to remove any solids.

Additional Tips:

- Feel free to adjust the amount of spices according to your taste preferences.
- Golden milk is particularly beneficial when consumed before bedtime, as it can promote relaxation and better sleep.
- For a smoother consistency, you can blend the milk mixture in a blender before heating.

Chamomile & Lavender Bath

This soothing ritual is relaxing and promotes all-around relaxation and stress relief. It helps improve sleep quality and nourishes the skin with anti-inflammatory properties.

Ingredients: 1/2 cup dried chamomile flowers, 1/2 cup dried lavender flowers, muslin bag.

Procedure: Place chamomile and lavender flowers in a muslin bag. Hang the bag under the tap while running a warm bath. Soak for 20-30 minutes.

Epsom Salt & Lavender Bath

This is another lovely way to relieve stress, whilst helping with muscle tension, cramps, and toxin elimination. An Epsom salt and lavender bath helps to relax and can improve sleep. The magnesium in Epsom salt is known to help to detoxify the body.

Ingredients: 1 cup Epsom salt, 10 drops lavender essential oil.

Procedure: Add Epsom salt and lavender oil to a warm bath. Stir to dissolve the salt. Soak for 20-30 minutes.

Herbal Foot Soak

This foot soak relaxes tired feet, improves circulation, and provides relief from aches and pains. The essential oils also have antibacterial and anti-inflammatory properties.

Ingredients: 1/2 cup Epsom salt, 1 tsp dried rosemary, 1 tsp dried peppermint, 10 drops eucalyptus essential oil.

Procedure: Mix Epsom salt, dried herbs, and essential oil in a basin of warm water. Soak feet for 20-30 minutes.

Calming Pillow Spray

The calming pillow spray promotes relaxation and helps improve sleep quality. Lavender and chamomile essential oils are known for their soothing and stress-relieving properties.

Ingredients: 1/2 cup distilled water, 1 tsp witch hazel, 10 drops lavender essential oil, 5 drops chamomile essential oil.

Procedure: Combine all ingredients in a spray bottle. Shake well before use. Spray lightly on pillow before bedtime.

Ginkgo Biloba Tea

This uplifting blend is renowned for enhancing cerebral blood flow, improving focus and memory, and aiding in cognitive function.

Ingredients: 1 tsp dried ginkgo biloba leaves, 1 cup boiling water.

Procedure: Steep ginkgo biloba leaves in boiling water for 10 minutes. Strain and drink.

Maca Smoothie

One of the great things about smoothies is that you can add as many delicious and nutritious ingredients as you please! This is a favorite, as maca (also known as Lepidium meyenii or Ginseng) is known for boosting energy and endurance, improving mood, and helping with stress management – a perfect base blend to thrive through our busy days.

Ingredients: 1 tbsp maca powder, 1 banana, 1 cup almond milk, a handful of spinach.

Procedure: Blend all ingredients until smooth.

Peppermint and Rosemary Oil Diffuser

This one is so easy to prepare and particularly beneficial when used in a work or artistic space. Inhalation of peppermint and rosemary oils improves concentration, memory, and mental clarity. If time-poor, you might choose to purchase quality essential oils and create your own combinations. Otherwise, steam distillation is an effective method of extraction.

Ingredients: 5 drops peppermint essential oil, 5 drops rosemary essential oil, water for diffuser.

Procedure: Add essential oils to water in a diffuser.

Lion's Mane Mushroom Elixir

This powerful elixir can be purchased ready to be consumed, created from Lion's Mane powder, or made as a tincture from scratch. Within its range of mental and physical benefits, it has been found to promote nerve growth, support cognitive functions, and help maintain mental focus.

Option 1

Ingredients: 1 tsp Lion's Mane mushroom powder, 1 cup hot water, 1 tsp honey.

Procedure: Mix Lion's Mane powder and honey in hot water.

Option 2

Ingredients: Water, 1/2 lemon, turmeric powder, fresh ginger, Lion's Mane extract, cayenne pepper, sea salt.

Procedure: Add filtered water to a large mason jar. Squeeze in the juice of the lemon half. Add in turmeric powder, diced ginger, Lion's Mane extract, cayenne pepper and sea salt. Fasten the lid on the jar and shake vigorously to combine all ingredients.

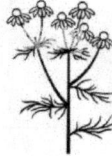

CONCLUSION

As we conclude our enlightening journey through this herbal healing handbook, I want to take a moment to reflect on the path we've traversed together.

From the very first page, we've explored the fundamentals of biohacking for women, unearthed the magic of plants, learned to craft our own remedies, and discovered just how powerful nature can be in supporting our well-being. Whether you came here looking for a way to ease stress, boost your immune system, or just feel more in tune with your body, I hope this book has left you feeling empowered, inspired, and maybe just a *little* bit like an herbalist-in-the-making.

But this isn't the end of your herbal journey. Not even close. It's just the beginning.

The beauty of herbal medicine is that it is always evolving. There is always something new to learn, a new plant to discover, a new remedy to try. Maybe today it's a soothing lavender tea before bed, and next month, a homemade elderberry syrup that keeps your whole family healthy through flu season. The key is to *keep going*. Keep experimenting. Keep listening to your body. And most importantly, keep trusting that nature has your back.

I also encourage you to connect with the larger herbal community, whether that means finding a local herbalist, joining an online group, or simply swapping remedies with a friend over a cup of tea. The wisdom of herbal healing has been passed down for generations, and the more we share, the more we all benefit.

And let's not forget the bigger picture. The more we embrace these natural remedies, the more we help shift the world toward a future where herbal medicine is recognized, respected, and accessible to all. Imagine a world where self-care doesn't just mean expensive spa days, but also a well-stocked herbal pantry filled with nature's best remedies. That's the kind of world I want to live in.

So, thank you. Truly. For being here, for being curious, and for taking the time to invest in your health. Writing this book has been an absolute joy, but knowing it's in the hands of people like you? *That's* what makes it all worth it.

Now go forth, brew some tea, tincture some herbs, and embrace the green, thriving, beautifully holistic life that's waiting for you.

Wishing you health, balance, and an apothecary full of herbal goodness.

Bonus Round: Where the Real Magic Happens

Congratulations, wise woman, you've officially crossed the final chapter—but trust me, this is where things get *deliciously practical*. Because knowing is only half the magic; *doing* is what transforms our health and rewrites our story.

In this special bonus section, I'll hand over some tools, tips, tracker starters, rituals, and shortcuts to actually *live* what you've learned. Think of this as a short and sweet herbal biohacker's version of a really good spice rack: organized, powerful, and designed to make every day better.

Herbal Hacks 101: Your Kitchen Apothecary

You don't need to be a witch (though we love a good moon-charged moment) to make herbal medicine at home. Here's what you might consider keeping in your toolkit:

- **Tinctures** – concentrated liquid extracts. Great for fast-acting support (hello, anxiety emergency drops).
- **Infusions & Decoctions** – herbal teas made with intention. Perfect for sipping your way to hormone harmony.
- **Herbal Capsules** – for those days when you want benefits without boiling water.
- **Powders & Blends** – throw them in smoothies, soups, or your favorite "I'm too busy" meals.
- **Infused oils & salves** – for topical hormone balance, lymphatic support, and goddess-level self-care rituals.

Sage's Tip: Start small. Pick 3 herbs you love and learn them deeply. You'll build a relationship with them, and that's where the real medicine begins.

Symptom Tracker & Cycle Syncing Pages

Whether you're still cycling, in the messy middle, or waving from postmenopausal shores, tracking is a biohacker's secret weapon. Not to obsess, but to *observe*. To notice what's working, what's shifting, and where you're still feeling stuck.

Your tracker can include:

- Mood + Energy Log
- Sleep & Stress Journal
- Supplement & Herb Tracker
- Cycle Map (even if it's irregular or "retired")
- Weekly Wins (because we celebrate progress, not perfection)

Rituals & Lifestyle Hacks That Support Your Herbs

Because you can't sip tea while living in chaos and expect enlightenment.

1. The 10-Minute Nervous System Reset

For when your inner peace has left the chat.

Your herbs (especially adaptogens and nervines) can only work so hard if you're running on nervous energy all day. This mini ritual gives your body the signal: *you're safe now.*

How to do it:

- Find a quiet space (or at least a parked car).
- Set a timer for 10 minutes.
- Sit or lie down, close your eyes.
- Inhale for 4 counts, hold for 4, exhale for 6. Repeat.
- Let your jaw unclench, shoulders soften, belly rise.
- Imagine exhaling stress out the soles of your feet.
- Optional: Sip lemon balm or tulsi tea afterward to reinforce the calm.

Deep breathing down-regulates cortisol, supports parasympathetic function, and enhances the absorption and effectiveness of your calming herbs.

2. Daily Sunlight + Breath Ritual

A sunrise moment that costs nothing and rewires everything.

Many of the herbs you're taking are supporting cortisol rhythm and adrenal balance, but this ritual *amplifies* their effect.

How to do it:

- Within 30–60 minutes of waking, go outside (or sit by a sunny window).
- Expose your eyes to natural light (no sunglasses for the first 5–10 min).
- Take 10 deep belly breaths while soaking it in.

- Optional: Pair with a warm herbal tonic or infused water.

Morning sunlight anchors your circadian rhythm (hello, better sleep), reduces anxiety, and helps your body produce optimal cortisol at the right time of day.

3. Evening Wind-Down Stack

Because your nervous system deserves foreplay before sleep.

YOU CAN'T EXPECT valerian root or passionflower to knock you out if your brain's still answering emails or rage-scrolling. This ritual helps you *downshift* so your sleep herbs can actually do their job.

How to do it (start 60–90 min before bed):

1. Dim lights (or switch to amber/red bulbs).
2. Turn off screens—or at least switch to night mode.
3. Brew a calming tea (e.g., lemon balm + chamomile + lavender).
4. Light a candle or diffuse relaxing essential oils.
5. Stretch or journal—just 5–10 minutes.
6. End with a few deep breaths or legs-up-the-wall pose.

Slowing the mind signals the pineal gland to release melatonin, while herbs like passionflower enhance GABA activity—both essential for deep, restorative sleep.

4. Digital Detox Ritual

Reclaim your dopamine and your damn sanity.

YOUR PHONE IS NOT your life coach. Or your doctor. Or your best friend. Create some distance so your brain can rest and your herbal nootropics can actually sharpen your focus.

How to do it:

- Pick one time each day (ideally morning or evening) to go screen-free for 30–60 minutes.
- During this time, do something analog: stretch, walk, brew tea, garden, sit in silence, doodle, write a gratitude list.
- Let your nervous system *unplug* without distraction.

Chronic screen time jacks up dopamine and cortisol. Unplugging allows your herbal tonics (like rhodiola or lion's mane) to work without constant neurological static.

5. Joy Tracking

Because joy is the hormone-balancing superhack no one's talking about.

HERE'S A RADICAL IDEA: you deserve pleasure. And your herbs agree. Daily joy increases oxytocin, reduces cortisol, and rebalances hormones more effectively than caffeine-fueled hustle ever could.

How to do it:

- Keep a small notebook or app.

- Every day, jot down 1–3 things that brought you joy.
- Doesn't have to be big: a laugh, a flower, a good stretch, a moment of quiet.
- Bonus: note which herbs you used that day and how you felt. See what patterns emerge.

Oxytocin—the "connection hormone"—counterbalances stress hormones. And tracking joy builds awareness of your needs, your wins, and what's actually working for your body.

You DON'T HAVE to do all the rituals, all at once. This isn't a checklist, but more like a buffet. Pick one. Try it for a week. Let your herbs support you as you layer in a lifestyle that feels nourishing, sustainable, and rooted in *you*. Biohacking isn't about being superhuman. It's about coming home to your body and finally listening to the wisdom it's been whispering all along.

Additional Resources & Herbal BFFs

Because every wellness witch needs a well-stocked toolkit and a few smart sisters on speed dial.

You've MADE it this far, so let's make sure you don't have to go it alone. Below is a hand-picked collection of resources, tools, and tried-and-true herbal BFFs to help you keep biohacking your way to clarity, vitality, and hormone harmony.

***

Herbal Tools & Supplements I Love

(Always consult your practitioner before adding anything new—but here's what's earned a spot on my shelf.)

- **Organic India Tulsi Teas** – Adaptogenic blends for stress support and gentle daily nourishment. (Caffeine-free and delicious.)
- **Gaia Herbs & Herb Pharm** – Trusted liquid extracts and capsules from companies with integrity and excellent sourcing.
- **Mountain Rose Herbs** – A go-to for bulk herbs, oils, tincture kits, and herbal DIY supplies.
- **Four Sigmatic** – Mushroom-based powders and drinks that support focus, immunity, and calm.
- **Organic Olivia** – Herbal formulas made by a fellow herbalist focused on modern women's health (with great taste).
- **Pukka Herbs** – Tasty, functional teas formulated by Ayurvedic practitioners.

- **Simplers Botanicals & Wise Woman Herbals** –
For tinctures with a more traditional herbalist's touch.

Books Worth a Spot on Your Nightstand

(Or wherever you read while hiding from your family.)

- **"The Herbal Medicine-Maker's Handbook" by James Green** – The classic for DIY herbal crafters.
- **"Healing Wise" by Susun Weed** – A feminist-forward look at herbs through the Wise Woman tradition.
- **"Adaptogens: Herbs for Strength, Stamina, and Stress Relief" by David Winston** – A deeper dive into the herbs that help you thrive under pressure.
- **"The Women's Herbal Apothecary" by JJ Pursell** – Seasonal remedies and rituals for modern women.
- **"Hormone Intelligence" by Dr. Aviva Romm** – Whole-body hormone wisdom from an integrative doctor-herbalist.
- **"Mind Over Medicine" by Dr. Lissa Rankin** – The science behind how your beliefs and stress impact your biology (and how to hack it all).
- **"Sacred Woman" by Queen Afua** – For women ready to dive into deeper holistic rituals, healing, and self-reclamation.

DIY Herbal Guides & Apps

Easy tools to keep you connected to your inner herbalist (and to help you not forget when you last took your tincture).

- **"Herbarium" by Herbal Academy** – A gorgeous, well-organized database of herbal monographs and recipes.
- **"Plant Ally" App** – Tracks your herbal use, logs how you feel, and reminds you to take your blends.
- **"Common Herbs for Natural Health" by Juliette de Bairacli Levy** (PDFs & digital downloads available)—Old-school wisdom still relevant today.
- **Pinterest Herbal Boards** – Curated boards with recipes for teas, tinctures, salves, and more. (Search wisely, check sources.)
- **Insight Timer** (free app) – Pair your herbal rituals with guided meditations, breathwork, and body scans to amplify results.
- **Moon Calendar Apps (like MyMoonPhase)** – Sync herbal cycles to lunar rhythms for hormone harmony and ritual timing.

Online Communities & Courses

Nothing's better than sharing breakthroughs, funny failures, and ah-ha moments with other women walking the same path.

- **Herbal Academy's Online Courses** – Comprehensive herbal education for all levels, from beginner to clinical.

- **Aviva Romm's Women's Health Circle** – A rich membership site full of science-backed women's health guidance.
- **The Women's Wellness Circle (Facebook)** – A supportive community for questions, herbal recipes, and success stories.
- **Nicole Jardim's Fix Your Period Program** – For hormonal biohacking meets cycle mastery.
- **Rewilding for Women** – Less science, more soul: sacred embodiment, feminine archetypes, and inner ritual work.

The real biohack? ***Trusting yourself.***

THIS BOOK MAY BE CLOSING, but your journey is opening into a space of deeper wisdom, sharper intuition, and improved well-being. You've learned how to hack your health with plants, but more importantly, you've remembered your body is worth honoring, listening to, and loving—wildly and well.

And just so you know, I'm still cheering you on. With a mason jar of hormone-balancing tea in hand.

Until next time, dearest reader.

Dear Radiant Soul,

Here you are, standing at the finish line—and what a journey it's been! If I could, I'd hand you a steaming mug of ashwagandha cocoa and a gold medal shaped like a rosemary sprig.

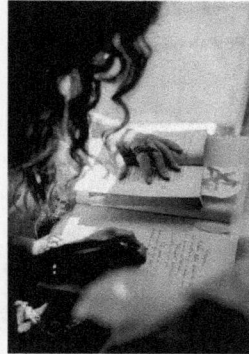

Writing this book was a passion fueled by women like you who are ready to work *with* their bodies, not against them. Women who know that true wellness doesn't come from a lab, but from wisdom, intention, and a little dirt under your fingernails. These pages grew out of a deep, stubborn belief that learning to biohack your health with herbs is both smart and soul-satisfying. And, if you can rebalance your hormones and sharpen your mind with a few tinctures and tonics, why *wouldn't* you?

So, I hope that you're walking away not just with notes in the margins and a few favorite remedies, but with a deeper trust in your body, your intuition, and the power of the plant kingdom to elevate every part of your life.

If you found value here, it would mean the world to me if you **shared a kind review on Amazon**. Your words help other women find their way to a healthier, happier chapter—and rumor has it, a little gratitude energy circulates back in mysterious ways. (Glowing skin, peaceful sleep, fewer "what was I doing again?" moments—you know, the important stuff.)

Sending you big doses of wellness, wildness, and a life brimming with vitality.

— Sage O.

Q&A WITH SAGE

Real Questions from Real Women Who Are Ready to Feel Like Themselves Again

---

Q: Where the heck do I start? There are so many herbs!

A: Start with your symptoms, not your shelf. Choose 1–2 herbs that speak directly to what you're currently navigating—like ashwagandha for stress, chasteberry for cycle support, or lemon balm for anxious mind loops. Master those first. Herbal biohacking is a relationship, not a rush job.

Q: How long until I see results?

A: It depends on the herb and your body. Some herbs (like lemon balm or passionflower) act quickly, within 30 minutes. Others (like adaptogens or hormone balancers) may take 2–6 weeks of consistent use to show up in a big way. You're not broken if it takes time; you're simply recalibrating years of imbalance, beautifully.

Q: Can I combine herbs or is that like mixing tequila and wine?

A: Unlike alcohol, most herbs *love* company—as long as they're aligned in purpose. You can mix 3–5 herbs per formula for targeted support. But don't toss a dozen random plants into a blender. That's not biohacking; that's herbal roulette.

Q: Do I need to take herbs every single day?

A: Not always! Some herbs are best daily (like adaptogens or tonics), while others work "as needed" (like nervines or sleep herbs). Listen to your body. It'll let you know when it's had enough or when it's ready for more.

Q: Should I cycle herbs?

A: Yes, sometimes. Herbs like chasteberry or black cohosh benefit from cycling with your menstrual rhythm or moon phase. Adaptogens may be taken in cycles (6 weeks on, 1 week off) to prevent tolerance.

Q: What if I'm on HRT or other medications? Can I still use herbs?

A: You can, but with professional guidance. Herbs are potent and can interact with prescriptions. Work with an integrative or herbal-savvy provider, especially if you're on antidepressants, thyroid meds, or blood pressure support.

Q: Can herbs really help with peri-menopause/menopause symptoms?

A: Yes, yes, and did I mention yes? Herbs like rhodiola, shatavari, black cohosh, dong quai, and maca can support mood swings, hot flashes, fatigue, night sweats, and libido. They're not magic bullets, but they *are* allies in helping your body self-regulate.

Q: What about brain fog?

A: Neuro-supportive herbs like lion's mane, bacopa, rosemary, and ginkgo biloba are the MVPs of mental clarity. They don't just sharpen focus, they support long-term brain health, circulation, and memory. And yes, they might help you remember why you walked into that room.

Q: I'm so stressed all the time. Is there an herb for that... and can I bathe in it?

A: Oh, honey. Meet your new besties: tulsi, ashwagandha, reishi, and lemon balm. These stress-lowering, cortisol-balancing beauties help you chill without sedation. And yes—you *can* bathe in herbs! Add calming ones like lavender, oatstraw, or rose to your soak for a full-body herbal experience.

Q: What's the best time of day to take herbs?

A: It depends on the herb's personality and your goal:

- **Morning:** energy, mood, cognition (think maca, rhodiola, lion's mane)
- **Afternoon:** stress relief or immune support (holy basil, astragalus)
- **Evening:** sleep + nervous system (passionflower, valerian, skullcap)

Pro tip: Anchor your herbs to habits, like tea while journaling, tincture with lunch, or capsules before brushing your teeth.

Q: Do I have to give up coffee or wine to biohack with herbs?

A: Not unless you want to. But be honest—are they supporting your goals, or sabotaging them? Some women thrive with one daily coffee. Others feel their cortisol go full beast-mode. Tune in, don't judge.

And consider herbal alternatives (like roasted chicory or cacao) if your body's asking for gentler fuel.

Q: Can I still biohack if I hate the taste of herbs?

A: Yes, my picky friend! There are capsules, glycerites (sweet liquid extracts), herbal powders for smoothies, and even herbal gummies now. You don't have to love every taste—but do find at least one prep method that feels like a treat, not a chore.

Q: I'm over 50. Is it too late to start biohacking my hormones and brain?

A: Absolutely not. It's perfect timing. Your body is constantly adapting, healing, and responding. Herbs can support you through postmenopause, aging skin, cognition, sleep, bone strength, and beyond. Start now. You're not winding down, you're leveling up!

THE EMERALD
S O C I E T Y

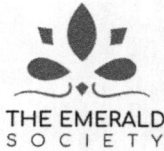

JOIN OUR TRIBE

Herbal Biohacking for Women

Natural & Ancient Plant Remedies for Hormone Balance, Mental Clarity, Stress Reduction, Immune Support and Graceful Aging

BIBLIOGRAPHY

- *Herbal Medicine* https://www.ncbi.nlm.nih.gov/books/NBK92773/
- *Herbal Medicine Today: Clinical and Research Issues - PMC* https://www.ncbi.nlm.nih.gov/pmc/articles/PMC2206236/
- *How to Choose High Quality Herbs and Herbal Remedies* https://bloominstitute.ca/how-to-choose-high-quality-herbs/
- *Herb-Drug Interactions | NCCIH* https://www.nccih.nih.gov/health/providers/digest/herb-drug-interactions
- *Herb Gardening Guide for Beginners* https://www.homedepot.com/c/ai/herb-gardening-guide-for-beginners/9ba683603be9fa5395-fab901a017fe5c
- *Essential Guide to Growing Herbs - Indoors and Outdoors* https://gilmour.com/herb-growing-guide
- *When and How to Harvest Herbs for Medicinal Use* https://www.hachettebookgroup.com/storey/harvest-herbs-medicinal-use/
- *9 Basic Principles Of Ethical Wildcrafting For Beginners* https://www.outdoorapothecary.com/ethical-wildcrafting/
- *Make Your Own Herbal Tea Blends at Home for Pleasure ...* https://healingharvesthomestead.com/home/2017/3/5/learn-to-make-your-own-herbal-teas-for-taste-healthscience-art-of-blending-herbs
- *How to Make Herbal Tinctures* https://blog.mountainroseherbs.com/guide-tinctures-extracts
- *How to Make Herbal Salves* https://learningherbs.com/blog/how-to-make-herbal-salves/
- *Herbal Infusions and Decoctions – Preparing Medicinal Teas* https://chestnutherbs.com/herbal-infusions-and-decoctions-preparing-medicinal-teas/
- *Enhancement of Innate and Adaptive Immune Functions by ...* https://www.ncbi.nlm.nih.gov/pmc/articles/PMC2362099/
- *Elderberry for Flu: Effectiveness, Benefits, Dosage, Side Effects* https://www.healthline.com/health/elderberry-for-flu#:~:text=The%20bottom%20line,and%20efficacy%20of%20elderberry%20supplements.
- *Integrating Conventional and Complementary Therapies for Autoimmune Disease Management* https://www.rupahealth.com/post/integrating-conventional-and-complementary-therapies-for-autoimmune-disease-management

- *Highlighting Herbs and Spices to Improve Immune Support ...* https://www.ncbi.nlm.nih.gov/pmc/articles/PMC7815254/
- *Herbs for anxiety: Does it work? Plus 9 calming options* https://www.medicalnewstoday.com/articles/herbs-for-anxiety#:~:text=For%20example%2C%20some%20ashwagandha%20-can,signal%20processing%20in%20the%20brain.
- *The effects of Lavender and Chamomile essential oil ...* https://pubmed.ncbi.nlm.nih.gov/33454232/
- *How to Make a Relaxing Herbal Bath at Home* https://learningherbs.-com/blog/herbs-for-baths/
- *undefined* undefined
- *Turns out your 'gut feelings' are real. How gut and mental health are connected* https://news.llu.edu/health-wellness/turns-out-your-gut-feelings-are-real-how-gut-and-mental-health-are-connected
- *Top 10 Herbs for Intestinal Inflammation* https://www.rupahealth.-com/post/top-10-herbs-for-intestinal-inflammation
- *Probiotics and prebiotics: What you should know - Mayo Clinic* https://www.mayoclinic.org/healthy-lifestyle/nutrition-and-healthy-eating/expert-answers/probiotics/faq-20058065#:~:text=Probi-otics%20are%20foods%20or%20supplements,as%20food%20-for%20human%20microflora.
- *Herbs for Natural Detox* https://www.traditionalmedicinals.-com/blogs/ppj/herbs-for-natural-detox
- *Efficacy and adverse effects of ginkgo biloba for cognitive ...* https://pubmed.ncbi.nlm.nih.gov/25114079/
- *Comparing the effectiveness of chamomile and valerian* https://www.-mayernikkitchen.com/blog/comparing-the-effectiveness-of-chamomile-and-valerian-for-sleep-and-anxiety#:~:text=The%20chamomile%20in-vites%20sleep%20by,is%20lesser%20than%20the%20chamomile.
- *Effects of Rhodiola rosea and Panax ginseng on the ...* https://pubmed.ncbi.nlm.nih.gov/31149868/
- *10 Health Benefits of Turmeric and Curcumin* https://www.healthline.-com/nutrition/top-10-evidence-based-health-benefits-of-turmeric
- *A review of modern and conventional extraction techniques ...* https://www.sciencedirect.com/science/arti-cle/pii/S2468227623000443#:~:text=In%20the%20same%20vein%2C%20-several,extraction%20methods%20are%20gaining%20significance.
- *Phytochemical Screening, Proximate Analysis and ...* https://www.ncbi.nlm.nih.gov/pmc/articles/PMC4700722/
- *What is a Customized Herbal Formula?* https://mkintegrative.com/what-is-a-customized-herbal-formula/

- https://www.youtube.com/watch?v=pjbmb4JLBTY
- *Clinical risk management of herb–drug interactions - PMC*
  https://www.ncbi.nlm.nih.gov/pmc/articles/PMC2000738/